T0094145

Doing Dignity

HEALTH COMMUNICATION

The Health Communication series features rhetorical, critical, and qualitative studies projects exploring the discourses that constitute major health issues of today and the past. Books in the series provide a comprehensive illustration of how health and medicine are communicated to, with, and through diverse individuals and populations.

Doing Dignity

ETHICAL PRAXIS AND
THE POLITICS OF CARE

Christa Teston

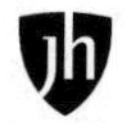

Johns Hopkins University Press
Baltimore

Printed in the United States of America on acid-free paper

2 4 6 8 9 7 5 3 1

Johns Hopkins University Press
2715 North Charles Street
Baltimore, Maryland 21218
www.press.jhu.edu

Library of Congress Cataloging-in-Publication Data

Names: Teston, Christa, author.
Title: Doing dignity : ethical praxis and the politics of care / Christa Teston.
Description: Baltimore : Johns Hopkins University Press, 2024. | Series: Health communication | Includes bibliographical references and index.
Identifiers: LCCN 2023029971 | ISBN 9781421448763 (hardcover) | ISBN 9781421448770 (ebook)
Subjects: LCSH: Medical ethics. | Physician and patient. | Patients—Psychology. | Dignity. | BISAC: MEDICAL / Health Policy | MEDICAL / Public Health
Classification: LCC R725.5 .T47 2024 | DDC 174.2—dc23/eng/20231213
LC record available at https://lccn.loc.gov/2023029971

A catalog record for this book is available from the British Library.

Special discounts are available for bulk purchases of this book. For more information, please contact Special Sales at specialsales@jh.edu.

CONTENTS

ACKNOWLEDGMENTS

It is only because I had access to time, space, and money that a book like this was possible. I benefited enormously from being at an institution that not only values research but that also provides the resources it takes to do research well. The sabbatical I was granted during fall 2020 enabled me to read deeply and attend online webinars and keynotes delivered by brilliant scholars such as Jane Bennett, Jack Halberstam, Anna Tsing, Liza Mazzei, Alecia Jackson, Katherine McKittrick, and Elizabeth St. Pierre, to name just a few. Two English Department chairpersons—Robyn Warhol and Susan Williams—continually found ways to guard my time and energy so that I could write this book. And without Andrea Lunsford's generous support via the department's first Andrea Lunsford Designated Associate Professor of Rhetoric, Composition, and Literacy, I would not have had the time to do this work.

Because of a grant I was awarded from Ohio State University's Global Arts + Humanities, I was able to hire and work with five folks whose expertise made chapter two possible: Melissa Guadrón, Shariq Sherwani, Goran Stevanovski, Ania Pathak, and Mahlet Meshesha (much gratitude to Robert McRuer for helping with the cross-institutional collaboration hurdles we encountered). Without the transcription services of Liliana Perez Rodriguez, Natalie Kopp, and Jess Vazquez Hernandez, our work together as a team would have been significantly delayed.

Thanks to Dana Renga and Ohio State University's College of Arts and Sciences Completion Grant, I was able to complete data analysis despite taking on additional administrative duties. This grant also enabled me to hire two amazing undergraduate research assistants, Olivia Andresen and Rheanna Velasquez, whose help was essential to completing chapter three. And for the email communication that helped me refine my thinking about so-called death-with-dignity, I am grateful to Dr. Jonathan Groner.

Chapter four of this book was possible only because of colleagues in Ohio State University's Assistive Technology Clinic—including and especially Theresa F. Berner, Wendy Koesters, Matt Linsenmayer, Diana Longwell, and Matt Yankie. Thank you for inviting me into your space so that I might witness care-in-practice.

Other department colleagues kindly reviewed chapter drafts and offered extremely valuable insights. Thanks especially to Molly Farrell, Wendy Hesford, Leslie Lockett, Brian McHale, Jim Phelan, Jake Risinger, and Amy Shuman for the gift of good conversation and feedback. The regular meetings among CareLab members (Addison Torrence, Ashley Tschakert Foertmeyer, Elissa Washuta, Emily Cunningham, John Jones, Liz Miller, and Margaret Price) provided fuel for this work in the form of care and comradery. CareLab was funded, in part, from a Humanities Without Walls Grant and an Arts & Humanities Completion Grant.

So many folks who work behind the scenes to help researchers get their work done must be acknowledged as well. I'm so indebted to our department's administrative manager, Wayne Lovely, and our amazing subject area librarian, Jennifer Schnabel. Sandy Shew saved my bacon so many times when it came to making NVivo for Teams do what I needed it to do. And Jacob Stoddard was such a fantastic guide through all things related to seeking institutional review board approval. My gratitude, as well, to Robin Jensen and Matt McAdam for their keen editorial eyes and support throughout this process.

I also benefited immensely from friends from the larger discipline of rhetoric and writing studies, especially Casey Boyle, Caroline Gottschalk Druschke, S. Scott Graham, Jodie Nicotra, and Jason Swarts. This project's analyses were made richer by the resources and ways of thinking and reading shared during a 2021 Rhetoric Society of America Summer Institute seminar, "Rhetorical Ethics in an Unjust World," led by Diane Davis and Nathan Stormer. To the anonymous reviewers of this manuscript: sincere gratitude for your incisive critiques and generous recommendations for revision.

Finally, I'm indebted to my mom and dad—Michael and Lois Teston—for their steadfast support, even if they don't always know what it is I do or write about. Thank you, Dad, for reading earlier drafts of this project and pushing me to say the thing academics mostly like to dance around in our writing: *We can do better.* And to my life partner, Christopher Elliott, thank you for reminding me to use the time, space, and money I've been gifted these last few years to rest and recharge. I love you.

Doing Dignity

CHAPTER ONE

Undoing Dignity

> Empathy could not find her.
>
> —*Patrice D. Douglass, "Black Feminist Theory for the Dead and Dying"*

One year into the COVID-19 pandemic, an image of the "hand of God" went viral. Spread across social media platforms were millions of reactions to a close-up photograph of two disposable latex gloves that a nurse had tied together at the fingertips and filled with warm water (figure 1.1). Wedged between the two gloves rested the hand of a patient who, because of visitor restrictions, was suffering alone in a hospital bed. The São Carlos nurse who used the hand-of-God technique reported that it was "a form of affection, stroking, humanizing, as if someone was taking her hand"; such a technique also helped her to warm the patient's "extremities that were very cold, the hand was very cold" ("Hand of God," 2021).[1]

News outlets characterized the hand of God as an "illusion of touch" and "love in a glove," while social media users responded with impassioned arguments to strangers about the importance of mask-wearing and about the need for equitable access to vaccines. Indifferent to whether the patient actually survived (she did), it was viewers' viral circulation of her suffering that elicited response. But sentimental responses "cannot address the institutional . . . reasons for injustice" (Woodward, 2004,

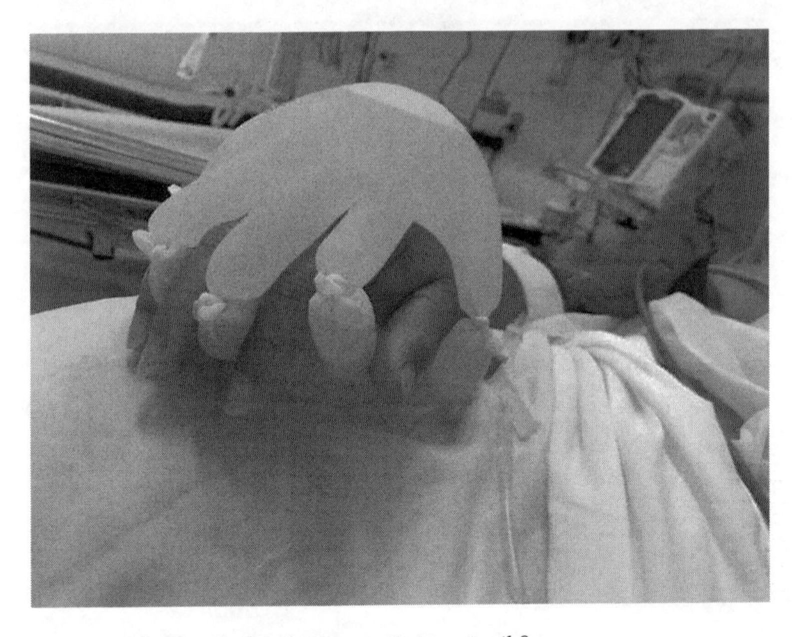

Figure 1.1. The "hand of God." Source: Twitter, April 8, 2021

pp. 69, 71). Sara Ahmed (2014) asks it this way: "Is a just response to injustice about having more 'just emotions,' or is justice never 'just' about emotions" (p. 191)? For me, at least, after the initial hit of affective despair wanes, what I'm left with is a kind of quiet nihilism. What can be done? Everything is collapsing. My sadness, anger, and outrage do nothing to change that. Me. I. My. Indeed, "Egoism mixes easily with compassion" (Lipari, 2015, p. 182).

I begin this book with the image of the hand of God because it illustrates what Wendy Hesford (2011) might call "spectacular rhetorics." The thing about spectacular rhetorics is that even as they provoke powerful emotional reactions, they simultaneously silence. Clickbait displays of sentimentalized suffering that purport to "unite us" through shared human experience—the experience, in this instance, of feeling cold, alone, or sick—obscure how the COVID-19 pandemic was (and still is) underwritten by stratified livability. Stratified livability is a construct proposed by Manderson, Burke, and Wahlberg (2021) as a way to index effects caused by "socio-economic inequalities, racial discrimination and uneven access to healthcare" (p. 2). As I understand it, stratified livability highlights how "some will—and some must—die in order that others may live" (Murray, 2022, p. 24).

So, while spectacular rhetorics explain why the hand of God went viral in 2020, stratified livability explains why, two years later as I write this, arguments for mask-wearing and obtaining COVID-19 booster shots are increasingly viewed with suspicion, if not outright hostility. The hand of God no longer inspires even a false sense of unity and compassion. Instead of receiving standing ovations, health care professionals in New York City are met with calls for the imprisonment of Anthony Fauci, the former director of the National Institute of Allergy and Infectious Diseases and chief medical advisor to President Joseph Biden. Much of the contemporary public discourse surrounding the COVID-19 pandemic in the United States proffers a romanticized, if not criminally fictional, "post-COVID normalcy." It seems not only that responses to suffering are selectively supplied but also that sentimentality has a short shelf life.

What is silenced in short-lived, sentimentalized commonality or "inclusion in some already constituted thing or entity" (Mbembe, 2009, p. 40) is how "varyingly vulnerable" we are (Niccolini & Ringrose, 2019, p. 2). Those who circulate hand-of-God imagery assume that bearing witness to an Other's (decontextualized) suffering will inspire behavior or policy changes. Yet responses to such displays of suffering involve little more than what are infamously referred to as "thoughts and prayers," which, of course, rarely address the intersecting power dynamics responsible for such suffering in the first place. Sentimentalized thoughts and prayers are a form of response rooted in an "emotional politics centered on empathy" (Oliviero, 2018, p. 237). An ethic of response(-ability) that hinges on empathy not only makes murky the material-discursive mechanisms that perpetuate the very suffering to which we selectively respond.[2] An ethic of response(-ability) that hinges on empathy is also unsustainable. Spectacular rhetorics' affectability waxes and wanes. Despite President Biden declaring in a September 2022 episode of *60 Minutes* that "the pandemic is over," it continues to have a mass disabling effect on at least one-fifth of those who have had COVID-19 in the United States (Centers for Disease Control and Prevention). What was once spectacularly sentimentalized is now normalized.

Critical health communication scholars are especially mindful of how the political normalization of human suffering reifies "cartographies of inequality" (Dutta, 2016, p. 17). By drawing attention to how health discourses perpetuate stratified livability, critical health communication research is situated at the intersection "of structure and culture" and examines how "values, rituals, and practices" (Dutta, 2016, p. 17) intersect with "materialities such as poverty, politics, and other social inequalities that limit people's access to basic needs" (de Souza, 2009, p. 693; see also Basu & Dutta, 2007; Dutta-Bergman, 2005). Such complexity makes it even more difficult to sustain an ethic of response(-ability) that centers on fast-fading empathies. And as critical race scholars explain, racism writes the rulebook for whose suffering is rendered legible long enough to elicit empathic responses in the first place.

Rhetoricians, extending Judith Butler's provocative question about when a life is considered grievable, inquire into how only certain lives (and deaths) are worthy of recognition or acknowledgment.[3] Black critical theorist and philosopher Axelle Karera (2019) responds pointedly to Butler's query about when a life is deemed grievable: "The 'grievable life' is determined by the color of its skin" (p. 51). To further illustrate racism's role in whether or when we respond to human suffering, consider Patrice D. Douglass's (2018) argument in "Black Feminist Theory for the Dead and Dying." In a section titled "Not *all* Women *are* Women," Douglass juxtaposes the "deblackened and unraced" Women's March on Washington against the silence with which Korryn Gaines's 2017 murder by Baltimore SWAT was met. Key to Douglass's argument is that "the specificities of Blackness are crowded out" by the "privileging of coalition as a unifying point" (pp. 106, 111–112). When Douglass asks, rhetorically, "Where is the march for Korryn? . . . Where is the support of her persistence? . . . Where is the march for her?" (p. 113), she's highlighting how sentimental calls for coalition are supplied selectively. It's worth noting, too, that some suggest that Korryn Gaines may have also been grappling with a disability caused by lead poisoning. Disabling effects caused by failing networks of social support (e.g., Baltimore's lead-laced water lines) are not always as legible as the "racializing assemblages" with which they intersect (see Weheliye, 2014).[4]

So, if sentimentality trends too spectacular, emotions too egotistical, and empathy too selective, what constitutes a "right response" to the human suffering produced by stratified livability? To answer that question, this book examines the in/efficacy of one alternative to "just emotions" (Ahmed, 2014): doing dignity.

Philosophers and bioethicists have for centuries tried to define dignity during caretaking conundrums such as those presented by the COVID-19 pandemic. Critics accuse bioethicists of thought-experimenting the life out of dignity, rendering it little more than a "theoretical sideshow" (Campbell, 2018, p. 1). In many ways, they're not wrong. For dignity to do the work we want it to do—that is, index a universal human property—it must be ambiguous enough to account for *all* of humanity. Dignity has, indeed, been relegated to the realm of abstraction. Rather than begrudge dignity for its ambiguity, some see its capacity for abstraction as enabling a kind of "conceptual breadth" (Debes, 2017, p. 9). Yet, the more an ambiguous and abstract dignity scales up, the less explanatory power it has for local moral quandaries structured by "poverty, politics, and other social inequalities" (de Souza, 2009, p. 693). As Nascimento and Lutz-Bachmann (2018) put it, "abstract values . . . may disregard particularities—such as gender, race, economic status, and others—that are often used to discriminate certain people as non-humans" (p. 7). Note how embedded, even in the latter half of Nascimento and Lutz-Bachmann's attempt to reassert the importance of particularities, is a kind of hierarchical calculation: to access nondiscrimination, we must adhere to a long (Western European) tradition of equating animality with abjection.[5] But shifting from abstraction to particularities while concomitantly clinging to liberal humanism's anthropocentricism does not rescue dignity from its vacuousness.

Dispensing with the heralded belief that human dignity is a metaphysical, inborn property of human being, Hannah Arendt (1958/2013) concludes that human dignity is "an intersubjective event of political experience" (Macready, 2018, p. 6). Inspired by Arendt's approach to dignity as both an event and an experience (but also troubled by what Mol [2021] describes as "the hierarchical version of 'the human' embedded" in Arendt's "theoretical apparatus" [p. 5]), *Doing Dignity* asks, How might dignity be *practiced*? Due to its capacity for unpacking how "practice" is more than just goal-directed human activity—it is, rather, an ecological endeavor—rhetorical theory underwrites this project's approach to understanding dignity as a practice.

Intellectual Spine of the Book: Rhetorical Theory

For those unfamiliar with rhetoric as a field of study, consider one rhetorician's explanation that, "contrary to its bad reputation, rhetoric is best considered a symbolic system that people use to make sense of experience and to persuade other people of the sense they have made" (Segal, 2000b, p. 30). Contemporary rhetoricians highlight how rhetorical acts such as making sense of and persuading others about one's experiences are not as discrete or bounded as we once believed. In place of *the* or *a* "rhetorical situation," therefore, North American rhetoricians now emphasize rhetoric's *ecological* nature.[6] Such an ecological emphasis echoes (and some say appropriates) Indigenous ways of knowing. For example, Manulana Aluli-Meyer (2013) describes Native Hawaiian epistemologies, which among other things emerge from spirit, space,[7] senses, "vivid interconnection," shared knowledge, meta-consciousness, and the inseparability of body from mind (n.p.). While (Western) ecological approaches are not always explicit about this connection, communicative practices rooted in "ancient and ongoing African traditions" are similarly ecological in nature. Moreover, Afrocentric approaches are "concerned with building community, reaffirming human dignity, and enhancing the life of the people" through rhetorics of community, resistance, reaffirmation, and possibility (Karenga, 2013, n.p.).[8] Rhetorics of resistance, reaffirmation, and possibility are especially instructive in my concluding chapter as I discuss how to do dignity despite being caught in a web of harmful entanglements.

Other rhetoricians describe rhetorical theory as especially useful when situations are murky or ambiguous (Hyde, 2006, p. 64) or when the future remains uncertain. That is, "rhetoric is the *seeking* of appropriate means precisely when evidence for the ethical distinction between what is appropriate and inappropriate is sorely lacking" (Murray, 2022, p. 13). Rhetoricians like myself who study health and medicine are especially keen to mobilize rhetoric's ecological approach to mining murky situations. In such cases, rhetoric provides for us a host of tactics for untangling and understanding how health as a discourse is shaped by experts, "lay constituencies," and a host of other stakeholders (Jensen, 2015, p. 523). So, while decades of scholarship has attempted to navigate dignity's ambiguity through deductive approaches that rely on historical, metaphysical, philosophical, and/or legal frameworks,[9] I see dignity's ambiguity as an invitation to mobilize the analytic power of premodern, classical, and contemporary rhetorical theories and concepts. Not only does rhetoric allow us to make sense of things that are impervious to "Cartesian rationalism, the canons of formal logic, and the procedures of modern mathematics" (Gross & Dearin, 2002, pp. 13–14); it also provides us with a vocabulary for critically appraising how things are going—that is, how dignity is (or is not) practiced.

Leveraging the affordances of rhetorical theory's critical vocabulary, I root this project's practice account of dignity in Ira Allen's (2018) understanding of rhetoric's charge: "The self-consciously ethical study of how symbolic animals negotiate constraint" (p. 4). For now, what I want to highlight is Allen's emphasis on the *negotiation of constraint*. In each of this book's three case studies, readers will encounter a great deal of detail about contemporary caretaking's constraints (which need not always be viewed pejoratively [cf. Boyle, 2018]). To develop a practice account of dignity, I am less interested in how health care professionals overcome these constraints and more interested in how they talk about and navigate said constraints. More specifically, I am interested in how contemporary caretakers attempt to carry on with the business of caring while simultaneously reckoning with the ways that structural inequities (or stratified livability) seem to render their efforts ineffectual. Such an approach allows dignity's definitional contours to emerge from rhetorical ecologies' particularities, or what Allen (2018) might describe as "a dynamic relation between constraint and possibility" (p. 235). Following Allen, I argue that opportunities for doing dignity emerge from the tension between constraint and possibility. In other words, in/dignities materialize (from) "specific physical arrangements" (Barad, 2003, p. 109) with which caretakers are perpetually entangled.

To study dignity is to study rhetoricity. Annie Hill (2016) regards rhetoricity as that which "incites responses, makes impressions, and produces effects" (p. 285). To Hill's definition I add Remi Yergeau's (2018) cripped, queered critique of the construct: rhetoricity is often theorized as a normative term that discriminates as much as it describes (pp. 178, 186; see also Price, 2011). According to Yergeau, some persons—especially autistic persons—"can never reach rhetoricity" (p. 46). In other words, one's rhetoricity and concomitant acts of addressivity and responsivity (Davis, 2017, p. 433) are typically predicated on white, male, heteronormative, and able-bodied logics of humanhood. Consequently, some persons are rendered "residual, lesser, and inhuman," thereby relegated to "demi-rhetoricity"[10] (Yergeau, 2018, p. 40)—a kind of "social death" (Hyde, 2006, pp. 136, 190).

The risk of social death can never be fully insured against since rhetoricity operates by way of what Allen (2018) terms human beings' "susceptibility" (p. 255), to which Davis (2010) might tether "affectability" and "exposedness." This book, therefore, examines how doing dignity involves not just susceptibility and affectability but also an ethical responsivity to an Other's exposedness.[11] Each chapter moves beyond hand-of-God sentimentality and decontextualized moralizing and draws instead on rhetorical analyses of real-time, ethically fraught contemporary caretaking conundrums. It's in the thick of these caretaking conundrums that the potential for un/dignified practices emerges.

Why "Practice"?

Due in part to my background in rhetoric and writing studies, my desire to construct a practice account of human dignity was, strangely enough, initially inspired by ethnographic research that reported on literate activity among the Vai people in West Africa. Scribner and Cole's (1981) *The Psychology of Literacy* marked a paradigm shift in the field for the ways it invited readers to view literacy as a *practice* rather than a possession that is or could be gained or lost. Concomitantly, practices are *communal* (Wenger, 1998). When invoking "practice," I am also highlighting "praxiography" as a method, which is the study of phenomena as they are enacted in space and time (Graham, 2015; Mol, 2003). More recently, rhetoricians theorize practice as adjacent to trans-individualistic tendencies; that is, practice is a serial, ecological phenomena wherein "we register an effect or register being affected" (Boyle, 2018, p. 53).[12] Important to this definition of practice is a kind of posthuman skepticism about what role the liberal humanist subject plays in larger communities (or networks) of practice.

In response to what some see as posthumanism's wholesale devaluation of human agency, *critical* posthumanism refuses to throw human agency out with the humanist bathwater. Following critical posthumanist thinkers, then, this book concludes by arguing for the revaluation of a remembering and reflecting self. Without the self, the power to both remember and reflect on the consequences of our "tendencies" (or practices) goes unrealized (Boyle, 2018). Critical posthumanists resist an indifference to difference by mapping not just "where differences appear" but also "where the *effects* of difference appear" (Haraway, qtd. in Boyle, p. 36). Throughout, but especially in chapter two, I characterize the effects of difference as un/dignified care both at and beyond the bedside.

To build a practice account of dignity, each chapter reports the results from one of three distinct case studies:[13]

- how health care professionals in the United States navigate a host of in/dignities at and beyond the bedside when caring for COVID-19 patients
- how end-of-life stories are more or less persuasive in public hearings on medical-aid-in-dying legislation proposed in two US states
- how physical therapists in a US clinic work with wheelchair users to find a good-enough-for-now fit

These conundrums, while situationally unique, illustrate ethical dilemmas associated with typified care situations in the United States at three different scales—global health crises; state-level democratic deliberations about death and dying; and intimate clinical interactions between patients and health care professionals. Each case study provides insight into how people in contemporary caretaking situations attempt to define and do dignity. Findings from my analyses help to identify, name, and illustrate (demi-)rhetoricity within fraught biopolitical situations.[14]

The book's first case study establishes the contours of a practice account of dignity. It sets the stage for the next two chapters by introducing readers to two key constructs: "bedside in/dignities" and "un/dignified asides." Excerpting from composite narratives from health care professionals who identified as having experienced caretaking dilemmas while working with persons affected by COVID-19, this chapter challenges discursive markers like "*frontline* health care workers" or "*first* responders" given the ways that twenty-first-century care work frequently involves *inheritance*. That is, as part of everyday, routinized bedside practices, care workers must adopt and adapt to several preexisting conditions, including, among other things, individuals' and infrastructures' preceding attempts at controlling or managing rhetorical constraints. Such (often failed) attempts at biopolitical control accrete over time as un/dignified asides. This case study traces how health care professionals' negotiation of constraint is perpetually stuck in a kind of existential pronation (the disorienting state of lying stomach down for COVID patients starved of oxygen) between in/dignities both at and beyond the bedside. Given the broader, infrastructural forces and failures with which health care professionals must contend, I describe how caretaking is as much "a political condition" as it is a set of "individualized experiences" (Oliviero, 2018, p. 26). As such, care workers frequently find themselves straddling the gray area between individual experiences and the politicized bureaucracies that structure said experiences. Setting the stage for the next two case studies, results from this chapter's analysis suggest that health care professionals are worn down by the seemingly endless expectation that they (re)invent responses to un/dignified asides or inherited "networks of relations of other humans and non-humans" (Rosiek, Snyder, & Pratt, 2020, p. 340), including human suffering, capital, commodities, and global supply chains.

Shifting from global health crisis to state-level politics of care, chapter three illustrates how un/dignified asides come to be mere "asides." How, that is, do state politics of care/lessness accrue over time in ways that normalize in/dignities? There is perhaps no greater embodiment of normalized in/dignity than public health policymaking. Building from the first case study's notion of un/dignified asides, chapter three illustrates how a host of local un/dignified logics of care/lessness scale up to condition end-of-life policymaking. The chapter examines public policy debates over proposed legislation to legalize "medical aid in dying," or MAiD,[15] in two politically distinct US states: Nevada and Connecticut. From these debates, I identify seven rhetorical patterns in contemporary death-with-dignity discourse, which I term "biopolitical *topoi.*" By cataloguing uses of these biopolitical topoi in public testimony, I unveil the politicized "moral predicates" that underwrite legal notions of human dignity at the end of life (Zemlicka, 2013, p. 276). This chapter sheds light on why some persons' end-of-life experiences are rendered "demi-rhetorical." Ultimately, my analysis of Nevada's and Connecticut's MAiD hearings reveals residents' troubling reliance on the pathologizing of dependency when discussing dignity at the end of life.

What, then, might it look like to practice dignity in a way that resists the pathologizing of dependency? Chapter four attempts to answer this question. In *Doing Dignity*'s final case study, ethnographic observations of physical therapy appointments at a local assistive technology clinic (AT Clinic) provide insight into how opportunities for in/dignity emerge during intimate interactions between wheelchair users and health care professionals. By zooming in on care-in-practice (Mol, Moser, & Pols, 2015) at the AT Clinic, I describe how health care professionals first witness wheelchair users' orientations to the world and then, through gesture, talk, and other forms of a/symbolic intra-action (Barad, 2012), they respond by *doing* dignity. Specifically, through rhetorical techniques associated with simulating, comparing, reasoning, recognizing, showing, teaching, measuring, and modifying, clinicians participate in a local ecology of care/lessness that creates the conditions whereby in/dignities emerge. Based on my observations of AT Clinic appointments, I argue that attempts at achieving what I call a "good-enough-for-now" wheelchair fit act as ballast against the destabilizing coexistence of bedside in/dignities and un/dignified asides.

Taken together, the three case studies exemplify how dignity is not an individual or even a social property of humanhood. Furthermore, doing dignity is not a choice. Rather, dignity is a networked rhetorical practice that emerges *in situ*—a response to our primordial "affectability or response-ability" to one another (Stormer & McGreavy, 2017, p. 13). Methodologically, each case study is inspired by a "microethical approach," which details how "individuals, as the result of contextual circumstances and ways of understanding, embrace different coping strategies and lines of action in relation to ethical values in everyday settings" (Örulv & Nikku, p. 509). Such an approach enables me to capture, as best as I can, the political particularities involved in doing dignity. One philosopher, summarizing Arendt, puts it this way: human dignity is "an intersubjective event that must be preserved and asserted by individuals and guaranteed and recognized by a political community . . . a *conditional* phenomenon of worldly human existence" (Macready, 2018, p. 7; emphasis in the original). In other words, dignity is "dependent on political action" (p. 7), yet dignity "may be asserted but not recognized, recognized but not asserted, or asserted and recognized" (p. 12). At the heart of attempts to assert and/or recognize dignity are, fundamentally, questions of rhetoricity. Who has it? Who doesn't? As each case study in this book demonstrates, one's rhetoricity is contingent on a host of entangled factors and actors that constitute the caretaking apparatus.

Why Do We Need (Yet Another) Theory of Human Dignity?

Whether in political speeches, promises, or international declarations, dignity as a construct has both connected and confounded us for decades, if not centuries. Recurring questions often bandied about include, for example, Is dignity something everyone (always) already has? Or is it *given* to us? If it is innate, how can it be taken away or lost? And to what degree is human dignity tethered to social status? Is it limited to humans only? Could it be that human dignity is just an overinflated synonym for more useful words, such as "respect"?[16]

Also puzzling is how often human dignity is deployed discursively in ways that are contradictory. For example, consider how frequently human dignity is used as an argumentative warrant by people who are on opposite sides of the same biopolitical issue—from abortion to what used to be called "assisted suicide" (more on assisted suicide's rebranding in chapter three). Even in the case of capital punishment, human dignity is mobilized as a form of principled morality both by those who wish to uphold the death penalty *and* by those who critique it for how it embodies state-sanctioned murder.

Said simply: Human dignity shape-shifts. And in a way, that's unsurprising. We have been trying to make it do too much for too long. It's no wonder that some have exasperatedly thrown up their hands and declared it a "useless concept" (Macklin, 2003, p. 1419). And while I am not necessarily trying to rescue or revive the term, I *am* curious about why or how it became so stubbornly ambiguous. What have interlocutors tried to accomplish by invoking dignity? How has it failed? And why? Because rhetorical theory teaches us that words and contexts co-construct one another, it seems reasonable to try and map how contemporary conceptions of human dignity are palimpsestic of prior situations. In the next section, I attempt just that. I unravel some of dignity's knotty material-discursive legacy to examine how the construct's very origins are predicated on "a logic of social organization that produces regimented, institutionalized, and militarized conceptions of hierarchized 'human' difference"—i.e., logics of white supremacy (Weheliye, 2014, p. 3).

Dignity's Harmful Biopolitical Ancestry: A Reductive Overview

> In order to get together, it is necessary to divide, and each time that we say "we," we must exclude someone at any price, strip him of something, undertake some sort of confiscation.
>
> —*Achile Mbembe,* Necropolitics

Contemporary dignity discourse bears traces of pre- to postmodern thinkers' attempts at theorizing human dignity, attempts that some refer to as "orthodox theories" of dignity (Killmister, 2020). Most historical accounts of dignity's orthodoxy begin with Cicero. But readers should consult Remy Debes's (2017) fascinating edited collection on human dignity for a robust historical investigation that, in a lot of ways, contradicts some of dignity's oft-circulated "platitudes," including the roles of both Cicero and Kant in modern-day conceptions of human dignity (Debes, pp. 13–17).[17] By beginning with Cicero, I seek not to replicate potentially inaccurate historical dogma but rather to describe how dignity's dogma has set the stage for a version of dignity that we must now work to undo. Denise Ferreira da Silva (2018) suggests (and I agree) that the "human" precursor to "human dignity"—which did not begin to appear until the end of the eighteenth century[18]—is "a racial signifier" (p. 25). So how did that come to be?

For premodern thinkers, dignity was a way of demarcating an individual's superiority or worth within a community. Historians, political theorists, and legal scholars tend to hold Cicero responsible for dignity's hierarchical quality. Ciceronian dignities conferred "a standard of virtuous self-command that is rooted in a 'superior' human capacity to govern passions and instincts" (Darwall, 2017, p. 185). What is important about this version of dignity's origin story is that dignity was fundamentally a comparative construct. Ciceronian dignity asks, How worthy is this person *in relation to* another? Dignity's Greco-Roman roots—in *hominis dignitas*—facilitated hierarchical humanhood, in other words. Contradicting contemporary thinkers who mobilize dignity as a warrant for equality and human rights (what Łuków [2018] calls the "founding-value thesis"), "nothing in the Ciceronian notion of human dignity requires, or even leads naturally to, basic human rights" (Darwall, p. 183). As many philosophers and bioethicists have declared, contemporary notions of dignity attempting to revive *hominis dignitas* ought to be cast onto the ash heap of human history.

By the time of the Middle Ages and into the Renaissance, dignity is rebranded as less a justification for caste and class (although both persist) and more as a divine mandate. That is, while social hierarchies certainly persevered, dignity was imagined as a God-given quality unique to humans among living things. Humans' rank, so to speak, was divinely installed by a holy deity. This version of dignity doubles down on human exceptionalism. Made in the image of God (*imago dei*), (some) humans were set apart from the "fish of the sea, the birds of the heavens, the beasts of the field, all the creeping things that creep on the earth" (Ezekiel 38:20). Contemporary references to dignity as "endowed by our Creator" likely have their roots in a theological understanding of humanhood.[19] This logic is especially prevalent, as one might imagine, among contemporary Catholic theologians who mobilize human dignity and "*humanae vitae*" in anti-abortion, anti-contraception, anti–in vitro fertilization treatises and in opposition to stem cell science, for example—arguments that, themselves, serve to rank-order some life forms above others. It is during this stage of dignity's development that we see the emergence of the "normate template" (Hamraie, 2017, p. 19), a normative notion of humanhood best depicted in the Renaissance by Leonardo da Vinci's *Vitruvian Man*.

From the seeds of the Renaissance's "normate template" emerged Enlightenment notions of dignity. Most historical accounts suggest that Enlightenment thinkers—predominantly Immanuel Kant—ushered in a version of dignity upon which contemporary Western philosophies of dignity are based. Kantian dignity, as the story goes, provides the framework for notions of autonomy and personhood rooted in normative standards and "harmonic proportionality" (Hamraie, 2017, p. 25).[20] In particular, much modern-day discourse about dignity tends to hail from Kant's "categorical imperative," which indexes a moral obligation to, among other things, treat others as "ends in themselves," never as means. According to Kant, human beings are without price. And the way to achieve such an ideal is to choose to make it so by acting morally. For Kant, then, dignity was not necessarily "an intrinsic quality of all human beings in so far as they carry the moral law within themselves"; rather, "it is a feature of those who follow the moral law's command" (Rosen, 2012, p. 29). Kantian dignity hinges on autonomous choice, in other words.

We see traces of Kantian dignity, especially his categorical imperative, in contemporary bioethicists' wielding of dignity to warn against humans' instrumental treatment of other humans as biomedical means to an end (e.g., human organ trafficking or medical experiments on incarcerated individuals). In essays commissioned by President George W. Bush's Council on Bioethics, "Kant" appears almost as many times as "God" appears (n = 200) (*Human dignity and bioethics*, 2008). Importantly, Kant's deontological dignity placed *a priori* demands on humans to act rightly, regardless of the situation.[21] Stoic philosophy took deontologized dignity a step further by emphasizing humans' duty to one another. That is, social bonds "involving all *men*" were predicated on human dignity (Griffin, 2017, p. 57; emphasis added). One might think Darwin's "descent with modification" and "natural selection" dealt the death knell for dignity's God-given human exceptionalism. But as Sylvia Wynter (1994) describes in her critique of the very category of the human, "the new Narrative of Evolution . . . of an *evolutionarily selected being*" simply supplanted the "*divinely created being*" (p. 48; emphasis in the original). Kantian reason—a quality available only to (certain) human animals, of course—fills the gap left behind by the destruction of the divine order. What emerged was dignity as a metaphysical quality available to (certain) humans with the capacity for reason. An "inner kernel." However, not all persons, such as those with cognitive disabilities, possessed such an inner kernel. Those deemed biologically inferior were, as Wynter (2003) describes, "dysselected" within the rubric of so-called natural selection. Contemporary discourse about dignity that relies on appeals to someone's "humanity" likely has roots in Enlightenment-era notions of the "inner kernel" and is, as Wynter (1994) argues, more of the same: rankings that "function to systematically predetermine the sharply unequal re-distribution of . . . collectively produced global resources" (p. 6).

Human dignity's origin stories rhetorically precondition the racism, classism, sexism, and ableism of the nineteenth and twentieth centuries through logics that "apportion and delimit which humans can lay claim to full human status and which humans cannot" (Weheliye, 2014, p. 3). Modern approaches to dignity are critical not necessarily of Kant's scientific racism but of humanism's overconfidence. One expert in ancient philosophy, for example, labels a whole class of modern philosophers as dignity "debunkers" and "saboteurs" who, starting with Schopenhauer, "discovered something incoherent, misguided, or otherwise amiss in the traditional concept of human dignity" (Calhoun, 2013, pp. 32–33). Troubled by world wars, fascism, slavery, and a host of other indignities, debunkers and saboteurs questioned the efficacy of a word that, by that point, seemed little more than wishful thinking. Schopenhauer, Nietzsche, Freud, and Darwin are just some of the many debunkers and saboteurs who took Kantian morality to task not just for its anthropocentrism (or what Morris [2020] calls "species snobbery") but also for the reason that "dignity cannot work in contemporary intellectual culture, especially in the light of the anthropology of modern natural science" (Calhoun, p. 34).

Embedded in skepticism about dignity's modern-day applicability is a marked shift away from merit-based notions of dignity and toward neo-Kantian, moralized versions. Martha Nussbaum's (2019) capabilities approach, for example, has "nothing to do with rank or status" and purports to be "profoundly egalitarian" (p. 70). And at first glance, it might seem so. After all, Nussbaum's non-metaphysical dignity can even be extended "to the lives of non-human animals" (p. 77). Nussbaum's (2008) approach to dignity is also careful to acknowledge how sociopolitical conditions affect how "capacities can develop and unfold" (p. 359). Yet disability theory scholars point out how Nussbaum's list of 10 core capabilities revives the "normate template" (Hamraie, 2017) through norms "of human species functioning" (Kittay, 2005, p. 109)—norms that serve to categorize disabled persons as less than human, even if that was not Nussbaum's intention. In a recent dissertation, titled "Human Dignity: In (Pragmatistic) Defence of a (Purportedly) Useless Concept," the author warns readers against "tethering our dignity to neurotypical capacities" (Morris, 2020, p. 9), which serves only to further categorize individuals along a graduated continuum of nonhumanity–humanity.

Today, neo-Kantian notions of dignity persist by lending moral heft to demands for human rights.[22] The Universal Declaration of Human Rights, which was flanked in the United States by (white) women's suffrage and the civil rights movement, pushed dignity far beyond its premodern limits. If all humans are legally recognized as equal—regardless of the mechanism that makes that possible (for instance, divine intervention or some humans' biological capacity for reason)—then they are entitled to certain rights. And if all humans are entitled to certain rights, there had better be a way to hold folks legally accountable when such rights are violated. Justice, then, emerged as dignity's kin.

This is but a brief and inexhaustive genealogy of how Western European notions of dignity shape-shifted over time in response to political economies, scientific advances, social movements, and human suffering. Now that the state is responsible for recognizing the inherent worth of all human beings, one might wonder whether "dignity is a relationship between people and politics, one that disappears when governments incarcerate and kill" (Debes, 2017, p. 12). Embedded in such a query is an awareness, I think, of what Weheliye (2014) describes as "a set of sociopolitical processes that discipline humanity into full humans, not-quite-humans, and nonhumans" (p. 4). In the next chapter, for example, readers will encounter a COVID-19 caretaking narrative from a health care professional who describes how one of her patients, "an illegal immigrant," needed a double lung transplant, but because she was in the United States "illegally," she was unlikely to receive it. Given such racializing assemblages (Weheliye), contemporary dignity discourse tries to get dignity to do the heavy lifting required of a property of categorization that is (all at once) an innate, metaphysical, existential, and moral concept now also modulated by a more extrinsic and context-specific guarantee of certain political entitlements. In other words, we've tried to make human dignity do all the work necessary to resolve the ways democracy's origin story is rooted in a "*community of separation*" (Mbembe, 2019, p. 17; emphasis in the original). Meanwhile, modern-day medicine hails from "ritual violence" (Murray, 2022, p. 26). Human dignity, then, often gets wielded as an attempt to plaster over centuries of hierarchical humanhood: a "bitter sediment" underlying plantations, colonies, and liberal democracy (Mbembe, p. 20). What is needed now is a "new genre" (Wynter, 2003) of human dignity that takes responsibility for such multiscalar harm.

Under the delusion that some mythical version of democracy might rescue the future from the havoc caused by hierarchical humanhood, a new brand of dignity has emerged under the rubric of "multivocality" (LaVaque-Manty, 2017, p. 308). Dignity's multivocality signals attempts to push back against Kantian notions of one-size-fits-all dignity. For example, multivocalists describe dignity as a kind of metaphorical balloon whose skin is a generalized understanding of dignity that gives shape to, stretches, and shrinks according to its internal contents, which are particularized "expressions" of so-called personal dignity (Pullman, 2004, p. 173). Others postulate that dignity might be more of an "attitude"—"not a fixed foundation for norms" but rather "a contingent good, that is to be reached or secured by a norm" (Weber-Guskar, 2020, p. 138). To examine its multivocality, some have attempted to define dignity by articulating its opposite, such as humiliation (Fukuyama, 2019)[23] or displacement (Mosel & Holloway, 2019).

Recently, researchers have investigated dignity's multivocality by using ethnographic and other empirical methods. For example, scholars have asked, What does dignity look like in "non-democracies" or places where women carry out "a host of the 'caretaking' tasks" (Nikolayenko, 2020, p. 465)? Empirical studies of dignity have helped theorists refine a vocabulary for discussing dignity. In a grounded theory study of dignity and health, Jacobson (2012) taxonomizes dignity according to two main types: human versus social dignity, each of which can either be "promoted" or "violated." Another empirical study of nursing care in a psychiatric hospital detaches *humanitas* from *dignitas,* wherein the latter is an aesthetic form "of sociality" that relates "to differences between people" (Pols, 2013). At their core, these projects rely on finding "ways to respond to a demand for justice that 'no right can assure' " (Davis, 2017, p. 434). Note that last part: *that no right can assure.* Rights-based frameworks for dignity do, indeed, have limitations. To mine that a bit further, I turn now to "communitarian approaches" to human dignity.[24]

Embedded in a communitarian approach to dignity is an emphasis on one's duties and obligations to others. Communitarian approaches share some affinities with the duty-based frameworks described earlier, which place certain demands on persons to (choose to) act in particular ways. Despite the temptation to see duty- and rights-based frameworks as kin, however, we should heed Motsamai Molefe's (2018) warning about how rights-based frameworks can "clash" with Afro-communitarianism, in particular. Afro-communitarianism prioritizes duties first and rights second. Here, Molefe is invoking Nigerian philosopher Ifeanyi Menkiti (1984), who states that "man is defined by reference to the environing community . . . 'I am because we are, and since we are, therefore I am' " (p. 171). Such an understanding of dignity embodies a marked shift away from individualistic notions of rights underwritten by presumptions of universality. Arguing that Westerners tend to inaccurately synonymize human rights with human dignity in an otherwise well-meaning assertion that human rights aren't unique to Western society, one scholar offers more nuance: human *rights* are core to Western society, but human *dignity* in Islamic, African, Chinese, Indian, and Soviet societies does not prioritize rights over communal duties to one another (Donnelly, 1982).

Importantly, communitarian duties are not framed as charity or compassion. Rather, duty-based dignity is, itself, the route to humanhood. Take, for example, the communitarian idea of *ubuntu,* which "refers to a human being who has attained a status of being a person" (Molefe, 2018, p. 225). *Ubuntu,* a notion "found in diverse forms in many societies throughout Africa," is "an ancient African code of ethics" that emphasizes "the importance of hospitality, generosity and respect for all members of the community, and embraces the view that we all belong to one human family" (Murithi, 2007, p. 281). Here, one's self-actualization is tethered to (or perhaps entangled with) the flourishing of others. One scholar describes it this way:

> In the Zulu language, the expression is *umuntu ngumuntu ngabantu* which translates as, "a person is a person through other persons" (Shutte 1993:46). Louw (1998), quoting Van der Merwe (1996:1), argues that another reading of this phrase is, "A human being is a human being through (*the otherness of*) other human beings." At the heart of *ubuntu* is a respect for a diversity of what it means to be human (Eze 2008). Van der Merwe (1996) argues that *ubuntu* is not just descriptive but also a normative ethical claim about how we *should* behave towards others and how to become human. (Berghs, 2017, p. 2)

Contrary to the autonomous subject, then, communitarian approaches to dignity are "*purely* other-regarding" (Molefe, p. 227; emphasis in the original). Kamwangamalu (2013) describes how *ubuntu* necessitates attunement not just to communalism but also to interdependence. To put it simply, a rights-based framework for dignity is "self-oriented," while a duties-based framework is "other-oriented" (Molefe, p. 228) or interdependent (Kamwangamalu).

Before (white, Western) readers romanticize (or colonize) communitarian approaches, it is important to remember the precondition for such approaches to be possible in the first place: trust. Trust is hard to come by these days, especially in modern medicine. Advocating for what she calls "epistemic humility," Anita Ho (2011) points out that "some patient groups carry certain social vulnerabilities that can be exacerbated when they extend trust to health-care professionals" (p. 102). This project's theoretical framework, therefore, is sensitized to how "power and status distort biomedical encounters" (Benjamin, 2016, p. 970). Herein lies the importance of doing dignity's "ethical charge," which is animated by an ethical (not ego-driven) self-consciousness. Doing dignity's ethical charge is "to determine what sorts of interactions can produce trust in a particular context," which "requires self-conscious attention to the power relations structuring that context" (Allen, 2018, p. 88). Although some posthumanists do, in fact, "balk at this emphasis on self-consciousness" (Allen, p. 103), I contend that it is precisely because of our capacity for self-consciousness (what Allen calls a "concretely negating restlessness of being" [p. 103]) that we're able to critique the figure of the liberal humanist subject that's caused so much trouble up to this point. Self-consciousness is, as Allen describes, a (perpetually dissatisfied) disposition "*toward* (always asymptotically toward, like the infinite calculus)" (p. 104; emphasis in the original). Without self-conscious ethicality, we would have neither reason nor desire to strive toward Wynter's (2003) "new genre" of human being.

Theoretical Framework of the Book

One group of theorists who are sensitive to how trust, power, and ethics intersect in technoscientific domains is feminist materialists (cf. Barad's [2007] "onto-ethico-epistemology"). These thinkers, including Karen Barad as well as Stacy Alaimo and Rosi Braidotti (to name only a few), refuse techno-optimistic, transhumanist enhancements as an adequate response to the human suffering caused by and perpetuating stratified livability. Instead, feminist materialists attend to messy relational entanglements. Feminist materialists' notion that humans are "materially embedded subjects-in-process" who "circulate within webs of relation" (Braidotti & Hlavajova, 2018, p. 8) echoes Indigenous cosmologies—cosmologies that long preceded posthumanism as either term or turn. Indeed, critical Black studies as well as decolonial, postcolonial, and queer theorists were the first to arrive at the scene of our "transcorporeal" condition (Alaimo, 2008).[25] As Deloria, Deloria Jr., and Wildcat (1999) describe, "The key to understanding Indian knowledge of the world is to remember that the emphasis was on the particular, not on general laws and explanations of how things worked" (p. 22). Critical posthumanists' emphasis on the particulars of relationalities also hails from what Walsh and Mignolo (2018), invoking Andean Indigenous thinkers, call *vincularidad*, or "the awareness of the integral relation and interdependence amongst all living organisms (in which humans are only a part) with territory or land and the cosmos" (p. 1).

In response to critiques that posthumanist scholarship is perhaps overly committed to decentering the human, Alaimo, Barad, Braidotti, and other feminist materialists, along with those who identify as *critical* posthumanists, are careful not to "argue themselves out of the picture precisely at a time when climate change caused by the impact of human civilization . . . calls for urgent and responsible, *human* action" (Herbrechter, 2013, p. 95). Diane Davis (2017) says it best when she confirms that *we* (that is, humans) "are the perps here" (p. 434). So, while feminist materialists such as those cited here hold humans accountable for harms caused by "globalization, technoscience, late capitalism and climate change" (Herbrechter, p. 94), the very category of humanity is viewed with suspicion. For critical feminist posthumanists, it is undeniable that who or what is deemed human hinges on biases related to "gender and sexual difference, race and ethnicity, class and education, health and able-bodiedness" (Braidotti & Hlavajova, 2018, p. 2). It is impossible, therefore, to theorize human dignity without (self-consciously) grappling with humanhood's hegemony.

Critical feminist posthumanists who critique the category of the human also work hard to counter posthumanism's reputation for failing to account for race "as a constitutive category in thinking about the parameters of humanity" (Weheliye, 2014, p. 8). To posthumanism's silence around race I would add a silence about disability.[26] Indeed, "the claim that identity emerges interactionally is incomplete if one overlooks the fact that not everyone can *access* interactions equally" (Price, 2015, p. 271; emphasis in the original). So, to make good on critical posthumanists' promise to interrogate biases related to health and able-bodiedness, my analyses are informed not just by critical Black studies but also by critical disability studies and crip technoscience. Echoing decades of Black women's critiques of the medical-industrial complex, Alison Kafer (2019), for example, notes how "medicalized technology is constantly being used to capacitate some and debilitate others" (p. 4). At the center of this project's theoretical framework—whether I am citing feminist materialists, critical Black studies, or crip theorists—are the tenets that technology is never neutral and humanhood is never natural. Human dignity's "human" is manufactured by and entangled with larger systems of power and so-called scientific progress.[27]

To summarize my argument thus far: Reimagining dignity as something other than a hierarchical, God-given, morally virtuous, or rights-based property of human being requires that we first recognize "the human's" harmful biopolitical ancestry. The next step is even more critical. We must resist the impulse, considering hierarchical humanhood's harms, to universalize, sentimentalize, and thereby flatten suffering. Audre Lorde (2012) warns us that "the need for unity is often misnamed as a need for homogeneity" (p. 119). Understanding dignity as both a product of and precursor to entanglements between humans and nonhumans, individuals and institutions, and capital and care requires sensitivity to "varying vulnerability" (Niccolini & Ringrose, 2019, p. 2). Critical Black studies, crip theorists, and feminist materialists provide a vocabulary for responding to varying vulnerability in ways that extend beyond sentimentality and even the liberal human subject.

As readers have probably surmised, wading in the tensions between thinkers from markedly different disciplines and intellectual lineages is at the core of this project. In his oft-cited volume *Biopolitics*, Thomas Lemke (2011) insists that "analysis of biopolitical problems necessitates a transdisciplinary dialogue among different cultures of knowledge, modes of analysis, and explanatory competences" (p. 121). So, in addition to my transdisciplinary approach to understanding dignity, other "friction-producing concepts" (Hamraie, 2017, p. 103) I use throughout the book are stylistically marked like so: "un/dignified," "in/dignity," and "care/lessness." The slashes are meant to signal a potential for harm that we can never quite shed because our rhetoricity is rooted in our "susceptibility" (Allen, 2018, p. 255), affectability, and exposedness (Davis, 2010). While I tend toward using cultivation metaphors in my discussions of dignity, I want to be clear that "cultivation and care do not offer control" (Mol, 2021, p. 100). Where appropriate, I also resist speaking of dignity in the singular or in a way that does not, at least discursively, honor its conditionality. As *Doing Dignity*'s three case studies will illustrate, in/dignities materialize through a repertoire of responses to and within larger entanglements of care/lessness, all of which remain in constant flux. Accordingly, this book's practice account of dignity offers a framework for ethical praxis rather than a moral mandate for medicalized notions of respect.

Methodologically, I take a rhetorical ecological approach. This approach allows me to unspool how humans' responsivity to complex contexts of care/lessness give rise to the particulars of doing in/dignity. But such an approach is hardly infallible: "The challenge of an analytics of biopolitics consists precisely in presenting it as part of a greater context" (Lemke, 2011, p. 121). Throughout, therefore, I try to remain as transparent as possible when describing how I arrived at the conclusions I draw. And where possible, I signal to readers where they can locate evidence I analyzed so that they too might try their hand at analysis.

Overview of the Book

The first case study, presented in chapter two, "COVID-19 Caretaking: In/dignity at and beyond the Bedside," begins broadly by examining how certain persons' biopolitical disposability is structurally conditioned. Given the consequences of human and nonhuman resource shortages during the COVID-19 pandemic, or what I call "un/dignified asides," this chapter illustrates how contemporary caretaking can be debilitatingly complex. Based on survey data, interview and focus group transcripts, and narratives from health care workers' reflective writing, chapter two describes how health care professionals (n = 109) grapple with bedside in/dignities and un/dignified asides in precarious conditions. As nightly news stories during the pandemic illustrated, health care professionals frequently employed creative workarounds to provide care—for example, by refashioning personal protective equipment so that patients could better see and hear them, leveraging the affordances of digital media to connect patients to family members while maintaining social distancing, and practicing other forms of "conflict-solving dignity work" (Örulv & Nikku, 2007, p. 510). Nightly feel-good news clips that romanticized the compassionate health care professional tended not to highlight the dynamic entanglement of human and infrastructural failures that had hastened the spread of the highly contagious SARS-CoV-2 virus. This chapter highlights health care professionals' weariness from continually being asked to respond to a host of inherited infrastructural failures.

One of the many inherited infrastructural failures that health care professionals grapple with manifests itself in public policy. Accordingly, chapter three, "Death-with-Dignity's Biopolitical *Topoi*," scales downward from a worldwide crisis to analyze two states' legislative hearings on statutory protections for a patient's right to die. At time of writing, only 10 states in the United States had passed some form of death-with-dignity legislation that protects physicians from prosecution should they medically assist a patient with one or more "life-limiting conditions" in hastening their death. The material-discursive evolution of death-with-dignity (from euthanasia to physician-assisted suicide) is a kind of rhetorical palimpsest for the complex network of capitalism, ableism, and racism at work in US health care policy deliberations. I analyze testimony from these deliberations to taxonomize—from two politically distinctive US states, Nevada and Connecticut—logics that underwrite support for or opposition to "medical aid in dying," or MAiD, legislation. This chapter describes logics of care/lessness, which are "mediating rhetorical and material elements" (Asen, 2010, p. 129) with different consequences for who may, and how they may, choose to die. To illustrate how logics of care/lessness have differential effects on certain bodies, I report analyses of video data and transcripts from the last five years of Health and Human Services committee meetings in Nevada and Connecticut, where MAiD legislation is, at time of writing, still under consideration. By untangling the network of biopolitical topoi (or argumentative premises) that structure un/dignified care at the end of life, chapter three details how contemporary dignity discourse relies on "pathologized dependency" (Oliviero, 2018), which frames some persons as more biopolitically disposable than others.

In her ethnographies of both telecare and contemporary nurses' foot-washing practices, empirical philosopher Jeannette Pols (2013) argues that "care practices are . . . material parables for moral questions that may emerge in societies where people give and receive care and negotiate about matters of dignity" (p. 188). Inspired by Pols's lifetime of work in and around care-in-practice, chapter four, "Embodied Dignities in an Assistive Technology Clinic," involves yet another rotation of the analytic turret to zoom in on real-time care practices observed *in situ*. How do health care professionals provide care to persons who have been politically and rhetorically rendered "disposable"? To answer this question, I draw on ethnographic observations at a hospital's assistive technology clinic (AT Clinic) to illustrate care-in-practice's conditionality. I extend Pols's project through a case study of how in/dignities emerged in the AT Clinic from what feminist science studies calls "bodying." Bodying is a rhetorical practice that indexes how humans are "constitutively constrained by nature-cultural processes and relations" (Snaza, 2020, p. 182). To be more precise, bodying signifies our immersion in "a network of corporeal relationships" (Shildrick, 2009, p. 149). Under the rubric of bodying, care practices are always contingent. In this final case study, I locate how and where contingencies arose and were resolved during some 15 hours of wheelchair-fitting appointments in the AT Clinic. My analyses break down how physical therapists not only accommodated wheelchair users' mobility needs but also contended with (among other things) US health care's economic roadblocks, as insurance coverage for any type of assistive technology requires written justifications submitted to the client's insurer. Here we see in real time "how symbolic animals negotiate constraint" (Allen, p. 4). This chapter contributes to readers' understanding of un/dignified care by framing it as a matter of fit, where "fit" is a "temporary result in the process of caring" (Pols, 2013, p. 39). Through systematic analyses of gestures, movement, and talk, I describe how rhetorical responsivity and response-ability in the AT Clinic involved "exposure to exposedness" (Davis 2010). Along the way, I point to structural conditions that produce immobility in the first place (e.g., anti-fat, classist, ableist biases)—even among health care professionals whose efforts to find the best fit may be stymied by market-driven medicine.

Chapter five, "Dignified Care as Ethical Praxis," shifts toward a more hopeful re-imagining of a "new genre" (Wynter, 2003) for doing dignity by framing dignified care as a kind of ethical praxis. Specifically, I remind readers of and discuss how critical feminist posthumanists describe the iterative relationship between ethics and response-ability: "Ethics is about mattering, about taking account of the entangled materializations of which we are part . . . Responsibility, then, is a matter of the ability to respond. Listening for the response of the other and an obligation to be responsive to the other, who is not entirely separate from what we call the self" (Barad, 2007, p. 69). I extend this rationale to make a case for dignified care as a form of rhetoricity that, yes, facilitates addressivity and responsivity but that also involves what Davis (2010), invoking Levinas, describes as "a fundamental structure of exposure" (p. 3). What emerges is a model for doing dignity that acts as a corrective to premodern and Enlightenment era notions of dignity—notions that, as described earlier in this chapter, hinge on harmful biopolitical categorizations and hierarchies. Eschewing the desire to make dignity a moral ideal generic enough to apply to all situations, I recast dignified care as ethical praxis. By reviewing the characteristics of in/dignity at and beyond the bedside from each of the three case studies, I argue that dignity is a rhetorical practice, not an individual (human) property. Conditional, not intrinsic. Never exclusive, sometimes therapeutic.

Additionally, chapter five "self-consciously" (Allen, 2018) reflects on the project's limitations through the lens of Walsh and Mignolo's (2018) definition of praxis as "thought-reflection-action, and thought-reflection on this action" (p. 7). Specifically, the very idea of "doing dignity" runs the risk of becoming a romanticized, neoliberal replacement for eroding (if not altogether absent) systems of social support. I contend with the ways a project that celebrates the localized emergence and enactment of dignity may, paradoxically, further what some critique as "asking individuals and local institutions to take up the obligation to ameliorate the suffering that used to be addressed by the state" (Berlant, 2004, p. 3). Within such a neoliberal framework, dignity as ethical praxis could be seen as a sterilized version of care that fails to contend with structural injustices that scholars in critical health communication have written about for decades. I end the book by reiterating the necessity of our ongoing struggle to shed liberal humanism's harmful biopolitical legacy. That is, before dignity can be done, its paradoxes—rooted in its meritocratic and/or hyper-individualized premises—must be undone. And as Mbembe (2019) writes, "No struggle occurs that does not perforce entail the breaking apart of old cultural sedimentations" (p. 141).

A final note before moving on to the case studies: In the pages to follow, readers will not find a prescription for how to do dignity. After all, such an attempt would fall into the trap of what Stuart J. Murray (2022) critiques as "affirmative biopolitics" (p. 13). Rather, again following Murray, this project is primarily concerned with the self-conscious interrogation of extant un/dignified practices—not proposing "new norms" (p. 13). Always a step behind, then, dignified care requires reflecting on a past only some of us have the privilege to forget. This is and will continue to be painstaking work.

CHAPTER TWO

COVID-19 Caretaking

In/dignity at and beyond the Bedside

> But then, when they start to decline a little more, their oxygen needs are increased. That's when we start to do more proning if we can. But some of those patients, they refuse to be proned. They don't want to be prone. It's an uncomfortable position to be in, especially for the first fifteen to twenty minutes. That's approximately how long I believe [it] takes for someone to kinda feel the full effect and be a little more comfortable with that position.
>
> —*Focus Group Participant, 12/14/2020*

When patients are prone, they lie in a hospital bed, naked, with their face pointed downward at the floor and their back toward the ceiling. The idea is that by turning an oxygen-starved patient from their back onto their stomach, pressure is relieved from the proned patient's lungs, and oxygenation can improve. Once prone, the lungs' delicate air sacs, or microscopic alveoli, unfurl and can better filter oxygen as it comes in and carbon dioxide as it goes out (Gröndahl, Jacobs, & Buchanan, 2020). Proning as a practice didn't emerge because of the COVID-19 pandemic. But as patients presented with a common COVID-19 complication called acute respiratory distress syndrome, proning increased exponentially.

The practice of proning came up in conversation only a handful of times among the 109 health care providers (HCPs) who participated in this case study. And it was never the actual subject of the conversation. Rather, proning was mentioned in passing or on the way to telling a story about some other care-related activity or event. But for me, proning was novel. Shocking almost. And at first, counterintuitive. Yet the HCPs I interviewed seemed to regard it almost as annoyingly uneventful. It wasn't until I started to research proning on my own that I came to appreciate its significance. First, it can take up to six or seven HCPs to prone a patient.[1] And because of the risk of accidentally dislodging the tubes, lines, and drains that patients rely on for sustenance, sedation, and oxygen, there's a rigorous, step-by-step protocol that HCPs must follow while moving in perfect synchrony with one another. Given its complexity, such a protocol can take up to 20 minutes to complete. Proning is time-consuming, labor-intensive, and potentially lifesaving.

Phenomenologically, the *experience of being prone* informs my interpretation of HCPs' caretaking narratives about patient experiences during COVID-19. In a way, proning metonymically indexes pandemic patienthood. Whether you are sedated or alert, proning requires that you be corporeally compliant in the moments leading up to, during, and after being turned. Having been proned, you are forced to reorient to the world psychologically and spatially in ways that feel unfamiliar, uncomfortable, and sensorially overwhelming. While literally suspended in space, you now see before you what had been below you. You are exceptionally exposed. Vulnerable. But (finally) able to oxygenate sufficiently, albeit uncomfortably. HCPs who enter the room are, for now, faceless actors. While swirls of activity continue both behind and around you, you are still. Stuck, if not unconscious. Your "bodily existence is caught up in material agencies that are difficult to discern, and impossible to escape" (Alaimo, 2016, p. 174). The bony parts of your legs and arms make virgin contact with surfaces they're unaccustomed to. Life depends on your acquiescence.

As one of the more routinized yet risky practices that HCPs perform, the *practice of proning*, as I see it, is an apt framework for understanding how in/dignities emerge during COVID-19 caretaking. For the HCPs who are doing the turning, there's little room for anything but absolute precision and cooperation. Done correctly, every step in the proning protocol is perfectly coordinated, not just between HCPs on the proning team

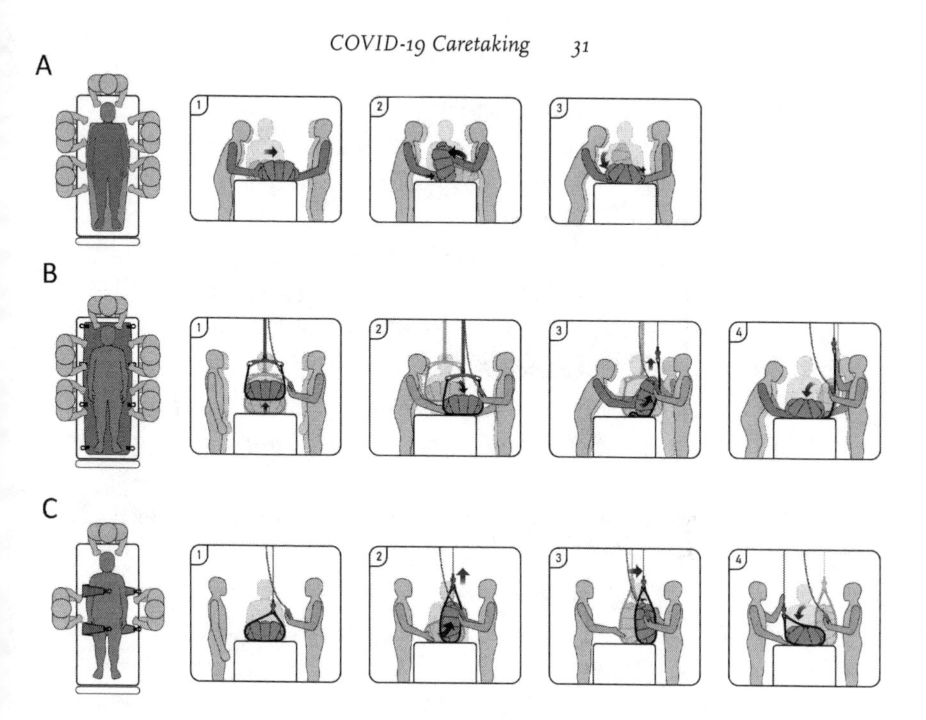

Figure 2.1. Proning a patient. Source: Wiggermann, Zhou, and Kumpar (2020, p. 1073). This illustration was created and provided to the original authors by Susana Peredo-Muniz

but also in concert with countdowns, tightly rolled bedsheets, and tubes, lines, and drains. For the person being turned, once your head and neck are secured and the bedsheet becomes a makeshift backboard, your body briefly hovers before being shuttled sideways. As figure 2.1 demonstrates, you're soon balancing on your side. Before completing the full rotation from supine to prone position, the patches and monitors that were once on your chest are relocated to your back. A new bedsheet is unfurled, and then you complete the full rotation from side to stomach.

Once you are prone, pressure points are padded with pillows or blankets. To assist with blood flow, someone comes in to rotate your arms and head every couple of hours. Up to 16 hours later, the process begins again, this time in reverse, and likely with a different team of HCPs. Everyone around you and everything inside you is in a constant state of flux while you lie still, waiting for time and gravity to do their thing.

Proning is, all at once, an experience, practice, and process that requires working with and against an invisible gravitational force. Certain tools and techniques can make the proning protocol smoother and more expedient. But comfort seems impossible. All involved begrudgingly endure proning as a means to an end. Inspired by proning, I've organized this chapter according to what I see as coterminous caretaking orientations—a "hung dialectic" (Allen, 2018, p. 65) between bedside in/dignities and un/dignified asides. I argue that HCPs, clients, and patients, indeed the whole COVID-19 caretaking apparatus,[2] are prone; that is, they are forced to both temporarily occupy and routinely pivot between in/dignities at the bedside and a host of institutional and infrastructural un/dignified asides.

Throughout, I use "bedside" as a kind of practical and intellectual anchor for analyses. "Bedside" both figuratively (and occasionally, literally) indexes real-time activities that occur between two or more actors who share the same physical (and, in this chapter, virtual) space. But while COVID-19 HCPs and their patients are grappling with what is, they must also reckon more forcefully with all that is or was adjacent to (or opposite of) what is—what I name "un/dignified asides." As a construct, "un/dignified asides" capture not just patients' preexisting conditions and familial backstories but also a host of other preexisting conditionalities—including racialized assemblages (Weheliye, 2014) propped up by infrastructural forces and socioeconomic failures.[3] Un/dignified asides are part of a "biopolitical apparatus" that "operates almost anonymously" (Murray, 2022, p. 23). Even as such forces and failures may operate incognito, working on and against us behind our backs, their dizzying effect reminds us of their consequences. Un/dignified asides may also manifest as "indifference and ignorance" (Brown, 2020, p. 119). In fact, Austin Channing Brown's description of "whiteness twiddling its thumbs" (p. 121) during moments of indifference epitomizes how indignities become mere asides. Bedside indignities leave traces that are "mostly invisible" even as they "attack the intangible (dignity, self-esteem)," while undignified asides' "banality" infiltrates "the pores and veins of society" (Mbembe, 2019, pp. 58, 59).

With the work of Weheliye, Brown, and Mbembe as this chapter's theoretical compass, I argue that patients and HCPs, alike, experience

COVID-19 care as more of a political condition than an individual experience (Oliviero, 2018, p. 26). Because COVID-19 created (and continues to create) so much uncertainty and anxiety about the future, HCPs in this study described feeling stuck in space and time, forced to occupy multiple, intersecting positions at once. Idris, for example—an older, Black, gay physician who began practicing medicine during the earliest part of the HIV/AIDS epidemic—frequently found himself relying on previous experiences of medicalized shame and stigma to understand COVID-19 caretaking: "There are many aspects of this COVID thing that are similar to AIDS. Here we are now, forty years later after AIDS, and we know that our newly diagnosed AIDS patients are still stigmatized. They're still limited in terms of health care. They don't have a vaccine. They have very expensive drugs." And like millions of other HCPs around the world, Luca experienced being both an HCP and a patient. As a giver and receiver of care, Luca continually wondered, "Am I going to bring this [COVID-19] home? What's going to happen if I get sick? Who's going to pay the bills? Who's going to do this [breastfeed her newborn]? . . . Like I said, there's so much unknown. We think we've figured something out, and then it mutates or something else happens. And then they find something else out. I think the fear of the unknown has certainly affected a lot of people." For all participants in this study, not just Idris and Luca, finding a way to (frustratingly) exist *in medias res*—that is, remain peripherally attuned to that which was and is, while anxiously anticipating what's next to come—was central to COVID-19 caretaking.[4] Forced to cope with what they could not change, HCPs had to acquiesce to a kind of professional pronation.

Initially, I was inclined to dismiss as overwrought tropes some of the phrases that participants employed when describing their COVID-19 caretaking experiences—phrases such as "balancing act," "slipped through the cracks," "gray areas," and "living on a knife's edge." But with proning as a kind of intellectual plumbline, I came to understand such descriptions as theoretically meaningful. The cracks, crevices, and spaces that light barely touches—the things that happen when no one is watching—here are where conditions allow for in/dignity to seed.[5] Before detailing how in/dignities at and beyond the bedside emerge, I introduce next the grant-funded Human Dignity Project from which this chapter's case study came. I also introduce the five HCPs whose stories are featured in the rest of the chapter.

About the COVID-19 Human Dignity Project

This study emerged thanks, in part, to a grant-funded project at Ohio State University called the Human Dignity Project.[6] To recruit HCPs from all over the country, I put out a call for a team of paid consultants who could act as key informants throughout data collection, including a medical doctor (Goran Stevanovski), health communication expert (Shariq Sherwani), social worker (Mahlet Meshesha), and student of osteopathic medicine (Ania Pathak). I served as a primary investigator for this project, and Melissa Guadrón, an expert in disability studies medical rhetoric, was my co-PI. In total, the Human Dignity Project collected COVID-19 caretaking stories from 109 participants via a range of methods: one nationwide survey (n = 109); semi-structured interviews (n = 17); focus groups (n = 13); and a reflective writing questionnaire (n = 13). All research materials, including the survey instrument and interview, focus group, and reflective writing prompts, can be found at https://u.osu.edu/humandignity/. Our choice to employ multiple methods was not just for triangulation but also because I knew from a pre-COVID-19 pilot study that, due to the sensitive nature of their experiences, some HCPs might feel more comfortable describing their work in one format but not in another.[7]

During data collection, which took place between October 2020 and February 2021, some HCPs reported feeling overworked and angry that they had been asked to reuse personal protective equipment (PPE). Other participants were frustrated with the way their employers and the US health care system, in general, were responding to the pandemic. To honor the way all participants spoke freely and anonymously about such conditions, I employ composite narratives as a method for retelling participants' stories (Saldaña & Omasta, 2022; Willis, 2019). Composites are made up of a series of narratives that, although combined, maintain fidelity to specific events as participants described them. Methodologi-

TABLE 2.1.
Composite identities of case study participants

Pseudonym	Description
Edna	Middle-aged white woman who has been working as a physical therapist for 10+ years in an urban area in the upper Midwest
Idris	Older Black man who is nearing retirement as a primary care physician; predominantly works in primary care in a rural town in the Inland Northwest; identifies as gay
Kai	Young brown-skinned man who just completed his medical education at an Italian medical school and most recently cared for COVID-19 patients as a physician in an urban field hospital located in a midwestern hospital's parking garage
Luca	Middle-aged Asian American woman whose work as a nurse practitioner has been erratic during the pandemic because of her own caretaking obligations and personal health concerns; works and resides in a major metropolitan area in the southeastern US
Naomi	Middle-aged Asian American woman who currently works as a hospice nurse but has extensive experience in social work; has spent time living all over the US but currently resides in a densely populated New England city

cally motivated by narrative inquiry, I dwell extensively in and then, according to common themes and patterns across their responses, relay participants' exact words by combining three to four participants' personal accounts into one composite narrative. Each composite narrative illustrates COVID-19 in/dignities at and beyond the bedside. Not only does such an approach afford anonymity for participants, but it also allows me as a researcher to condense a great deal of evidence into digestible summaries of complex phenomena. To be clear, while this case study is broad in scope, it is hardly representative of all US HCPs' experiences with COVID-19 caretaking.

In this chapter, readers encounter five composite narrative identities: Edna, Kai, Luca, Idris, and Naomi. Their names are pseudonyms and their descriptions are inspired by amalgamations of participants' profiles, yet anything I have quoted was taken directly from one of the study's 17 semi-structured interviews. Table 2.1 introduces Edna, Kai, Luca, Idris, and Naomi, whose stories form the backbone of this chapter.[8] The rest of the chapter is organized to illustrate bedside in/dignities and un/dignified asides in COVID-19 caretaking—constructs that I carry forward in the case studies described in chapters three and four.

Bedside In/dignities

Bedside in/dignities emerged *in situ* during routinized caretaking activities in real time—including therapeutic touch, draping and gowning, bathing, toileting, and other activities that participants characterized as "task oriented" (Naomi)—and were modulated by an HCP's "general bedside manner" (Idris). Throughout the interview transcripts, opportunities for bedside in/dignities were evident when participants referred to things like (im)patience with patients and their families, (dis)courtesy, (lack of) privacy, (dis)respect, (im)partiality, or (in)equality, for example. Edna described how important it was to be patient, especially when attempting to connect patients with family members, who, because of hospitals' visitor restrictions, weren't permitted to visit their loved one's bedside. She described spending hours helping patients who were "not very computer literate" connect via Zoom or Facetime. In fact, nearly all participants made reference in one way or another to the role that technology played in facilitating COVID-19 care, which affirms Braidotti's (2020) observation that COVID-19 has paradoxically "intensified humans' reliance on the very high-tech economy of cognitive capitalism that caused the problems in the first place" (p. 1).

Some of the low-tech activities on which bedside in/dignities hinged included, as Naomi described, "how to do a bed bath . . . covering someone, not exposing them, asking consent, explaining procedures." Naomi emphasized how important it was to recognize another's presence, even if they could not respond verbally: "Even if I'm saying, 'Sasha . . . I hope this is okay?,' and Sasha never responds, it's still important to give them that sort of courtesy." Invoking the Hippocratic Oath's directive to "do no harm" and the idea that dignity is "hidden in the idea of HIPPA [Health Insurance Portability and Accountability Act]" (Idris), several participants described dignity as respecting a patient's privacy. Naomi, for example, commented that it's easy to "forget to close the door when you're going to do care," especially when you've only got "one person in the COVID unit" and "nobody is going to walk by." Nevertheless, "you have to remember, no, I still have to close the door . . . even though I know nobody else is going to walk in there." Mol (2021) might describe such forms of un/dignified care as "tasks": "Willful and responsive, creative and adaptive, infused by desire and attuned to the circumstances" (p. 88). Luca provided a slightly different example of how the task of guarding patient privacy can be more complicated than remembering to pull curtains and close doors: "We've had a lot of transgender patients, and it's created a little bit of an issue for the staff and for other patients because . . . [i]n an effort to respect the person who's transgender, we have to think about, well, how do we, how do we place them with a roommate? What's appropriate and what's not? Is it appropriate to tell the roommate that your roommate coming in is transgender? Where are those lines at?" Because not all patients are what she called "mainstream," Luca described how she had started to modify how she asked about a patient's relationship with a visitor or family member: "And so I've changed my wording to go, 'So how do you two know each other?' And let them characterize it, describe it, however they want to." Luca continued, "Say I have a woman say, 'this is my wife,' and I go, 'okay,' and then they [feel like], all right, we can focus on what we're here for now. I think sometimes people feel that they are . . . I don't know what they think someone's going to do when they declare that they're not mainstream or something. But I'm there to care for their medical needs and provide whatever I can to help them through what they're going through. And I think that once people understand that, we can all relax and make sure that they get taken care of." Protecting patients' privacy was one of the many ways HCPs expressed attempts at doing dignity. But as Luca indicated, these types of tasks required tinkering: "The *doing* involved is iterative, it is of a probing, wandering kind" (Mol, 2021, p. 87).

HCPs also continually relied on respect as a condition of un/dignified care. In fact, after the words "patient" and "care," "respect" was the third most frequently used term among survey participants (n = 109). Like dignity, though, "respect" can be an unwieldy construct. Used interchangeably with respect was the word "empathy," for example. For Kai, empathy looked like treating patients "as if they were a family member of yours . . . someone's mom, someone's dad, someone's son." All five composite narratives alluded to how patients for whom the HCPs cared were someone's beloved, so they should be treated as you'd want your own beloved to be treated—*no matter what*.

It was in the "no matter what" that I detected a more nuanced sense of what respect looked like at the bedside. When prompted to unpack what "no matter what" meant, Idris described the following:

> Human dignity, diversity, disparity—all these, these *D* words that are buzzwords in the medical community today have become very relevant, you know, over the last decade or so, or actually over the last twenty years, really ever since the AIDS epidemic, where people have to realize that, that people of all cultures and all backgrounds deserve equal . . . equal, respected, equal care, even though they were considered marginalized populations. It's become a whole lot more obvious now in the last decade with Black Lives Matter and current LGBT issues that are facing everybody.

At the bedside, then, Idris was peripherally attuned not just to the Reagan administration's catastrophic mishandling of the HIV/AIDS epidemic in the 1980s, but he was also mindful of contemporary human rights violations in LGBTQIA+ communities and in communities of color.

For Edna, "no matter what" involved a kind of "impartiality": "having to treat a variety of patients, a variety of races, genders, religions . . . we as physical therapists strive to provide completely impartial care to any one person." When pressed for more specifics, Edna described physical therapy sessions with women who had certain religious convictions. In some cases, she needed to "switch people out if they got assigned to a male physical therapist" since some patients might "not want any males involved in their care." Impartiality also meant HCPs remained sensitive to religious and cultural practices for dress: "As a physical therapist, it's not our preference for people to wear skirts. But of course, if that's something that your religion tells you that you need to do, then we respect that and we work around it any way that we need to."

While on the one hand, HCPs claimed to prioritize impartiality, on the other hand, there were caretaking situations where *not* having intimate familiarity with the nuances of a patient's situation—described in the patient's own language, in fact—was an impediment to care. Idris put it this way:

> Sometimes patients want to communicate something to you, but there's a word in their language that they can't easily translate that to you in English, right? This might be an English-speaking patient that's bilingual,

> and they're doing their best to explain to you what they're experiencing. And then there's this one thing about their symptoms that they want to communicate to you, but they can only think of the word in their language, and they can't really translate that into English. And so, it's hard to really grasp everything that they're trying to tell you because you don't, I mean, there's a language barrier or cultural barrier.

While references to language or cultural barriers came up frequently, I'm not sure they fully capture the nuance of caretaking challenges in such situations. Being understood is inhibited by so much more than clunky or missing translation. In fact, even when translation was restored, the caretaking apparatus hardly seemed dignified.

For example, I asked Kai how, while working at the COVID-19 field hospital, he managed to care for patients who spoke languages other than the two he knows, English and Italian:

CHRISTA: Did they have translators on hand for situations like that?

KAI: We had the phones with the translator service on them that we used.

CHRISTA: What is that like?

KAI: Using the phones for the translator? Not ideal. It's definitely not ideal. It just feels impersonal to an extent where it's like you're talking to a phone and the phone is talking back to you and you're just looking at the patient in front of you, but it's tough to actually talk to them.

CHRISTA: Do you find yourself doing certain things to sort of compensate for that impersonality, or is it just like you're stuck in that situation and there's no way to make it better?

KAI: I think it's both. I think that you have to realize . . . You don't want to avoid going into that patient's room and providing the care they need because it's difficult to communicate with them. And I think there were, you know, there's people that take that approach. At times they say, "well, there's nothing I can really do in there because I can't communicate with them. So I'll just go in there if I need to for medication or for vitals, whatever it may be." But then that's providing a lower level of care to someone that again is probably in the more vulnerable group, just statistically speaking. So, I

> think you just have to keep that in mind. I know, I tried to, and it was difficult at times because you're taking sometimes fifteen to twenty minutes just to have a short conversation with a patient who you need to use a translator phone for.

Further complicating the awkward phone translation service Kai described was the fact that almost everyone involved in that situation was also wearing a mask, making it even more difficult to be both addressed and to address. Here's Idris: "We use a translation phone, but it's difficult because you have a mask on, you have a shield on, and so you're trying to speak to the phone and have them translate what you're saying to the patient so that the patient can then speak to the phone. But sometimes when you have a mask on, it's hard to, for the other person on the other end of the phone, say, to hear your voice."

Luca expressed similar frustrations with how PPE affected her ability to communicate, especially with patients who were hard of hearing: "And they can't hear you through the mask even more. And you're losing your voice, and then you're wearing gloves and eye protection, trying to start a line thinking, 'I could get this if I didn't have all this crap on!'" Seemingly aware that such situations were about more than PPE, Luca asked, "So how is that ok for the patient?!" Luca's exasperation expressed here was modulated not just by her experiences as an HCP during the pandemic but also by her experiences as a patient. Luca has a preexisting heart condition that, in addition to lowering her blood pressure, causes her "to get really, really sweaty, and feel like I'm going to pass out." While working extra hours as a nurse at the local jail during COVID-19, Luca experienced one of her episodes. Because she had worked in the jail, HCPs thought her perspiration might have come from contracting tuberculosis (TB) from an inmate. Fearful of contagion, Luca's colleagues "put me in TB isolation and basically did the same thing . . . They wouldn't really come in . . . [W]hen they came in, they had their whole getup on. It's just, it's embarrassing, and it makes you feel like there's something wrong with you, and people look at you differently."

At the start of the pandemic, Luca contracted COVID-19, and, since then, she'd found solace in an online support group for long-COVID patients called Body Politic. Not only did the Body Politic support group fill the gaps left behind by what some now regard as "medical gaslighting," but Luca also found other members' stories, or what Alyson Patsavas (2014) calls "cripistemologies of pain," instructive for her as an HCP: they had "really been impactful for me in learning about some of the things that people have experienced in our health care system," including being made to feel "like we've got the plague . . . [N]obody wants to have anything to do with you, nobody wants to be around you. Nobody wants to come in your room, nobody wants to provide that human touch, that human piece that we all desperately need." Luca's stories exemplify how bedside in/dignities are tethered to larger logics of care/lessness and abandonment, or what I'll describe later as un/dignified asides. Such logics "underwrite the devaluation" of Luca's long-COVID life and must be "exposed and critiqued" (Patsavas, p. 205).

Vulnerable patients' shame and embarrassment were common themes across HCPs' narratives, especially among HCPs who assisted disabled patients with routinized caretaking tasks, such as toileting. Naomi, for example, described a devastating caretaking event involving a disabled, incontinent patient and a state-tested nursing assistant (STNA):

> They [the patient] did not realize that they had a bowel movement, and when the STNA came in to change them, the STNA was very frustrated with them. The STNA wiped them . . . and showed them their feces . . . [a]lluded that this was annoying for them to be cleaning them up. Now, for somebody like my patient who experienced this, who does not have any loved ones local, doesn't have anybody coming to visit them, doesn't have anybody really calling them regularly, this can feel very isolating and very dehumanizing and very scary.

Naomi was careful to preface this story with a general observation: "COVID aside, it [un/dignified care] happens every day." Hers, in fact, was a common sentiment across all the HCPs: that there was nothing necessarily "new" about COVID-19's bedside in/dignities. "Honestly? The pandemic has not changed . . . how I see things. It just makes it more clear" (Naomi).

In popular discourse, we continue to read how the pandemic has "placed in stark relief" or "laid bare" inequities that have plagued US health care since its inception. COVID-19 caretaking, then, isn't only about what HCPs in this study witnessed at the bedside. COVID-19 care-taking continues to hover *in medias res.* HCPs and patients are stuck between, forced to pivot among, and must endure disorientation in a present that's already past or may never come.[9] Some of the stickiness that situates COVID-19 caretaking in a kind of existential pronation hails from a host of un/dignified asides.

Un/dignified Asides

Despite the United States' fetishization of the heroism conveyed by phrases like "*frontline* workers" or "*first* responders," HCPs in this study did not characterize their work as heroic. In their own words, HCPs described having to "meet patients where they're at" but do so in a way that required contending with a host of political, economic, and infrastructural inheritances,[10] which produce what I described in chapter one as stratified livability. As Luca described, "everyone has lived a whole life before I've met them." Others, like Kai, referred to such a disposition as having "a holistic view." Idris acknowledged that when patients "act out," it wasn't "because they're trying to make my day difficult" but "because of what they've experienced as a human." Mbembe (2019), when describing Frantz Fanon's "pharmacy," describes an approach to care similar to Idris's: one where "medical acts" involve being able to "answer the question 'What is happening?'; 'What has occurred?' " (p. 147). Again, some researchers may understand these utterances as empty discursive tropes, but when coupled with the stories HCPs told, attuning to patients' "whole selves" seemed like more than a new-age nicety.

When asked for greater detail about what was meant by "meeting someone where they're at" or attending to patients' "whole selves," Edna replied, "I think everyone's going through this pandemic differently. I think we're all in the same waters, but we're all in different boats. In different ships. Some people are in yachts and some people are in rowboats." Rather than yet another potentially trite sentiment, Edna's sensitivity to patients' "varying vulnerability" (Niccolini & Ringrose, 2019, p. 2) caused her a great deal of anguish. Edna described an ongoing battle with the fact that that "a lot of people . . . have a lot of things working against them." As a result, she said she felt "beaten down a little bit." In fact, many

HCPs in this study described having to make peace with the possibility that their COVID-19 caretaking efforts were unlikely to make a difference to the patient's disease. Whether because of patients' preexisting health conditions or a host of infrastructural inheritances, many HCPs spoke to a kind of existential demoralization, if not outright despair.

A significant source of HCPs' despair came from how patients' recovery from COVID-19 was in tension with their need to earn a paycheck. Here's how Edna described one of her physical therapy clients' return to work: "He's still struggling but doing better than he was. He's, I mean . . . [h]e's back to work. That was the biggest thing, that he's able to work full-time now because before . . . [h]e just would have to leave work and just take no pay because he just couldn't make it the whole day." Edna's hesitancy to equate the return to work with COVID-19 recovery points to a kind of unspoken recognition that capitalism and care are simply incompatible. Here, human being "is taken as manageable capital" where Edna's patient is "a particle within a system" (Mbembe, 2019, p. 179). It seems almost needless to say because it's so obvious, but capitalism is, indeed, a part of patients' "whole selves." Naomi explained it this way: "It's beyond just this feel-good thing. It's about structures of ownership, structures of responsibility, structures of accountability . . . And they all have to come together, right? You can't just have one thing. It's a whole new paradigm . . . And part of it is our relationship with the economic system and capitalism." To "meet them where they're at" meant that HCPs had to remain responsive to patients' financial livelihoods, which, of course, exist within larger economic structures. Doing dignity, then, is "distributed over a stretched-out, historically dispersed, socio-material collective" (Mol, 2021, p. 93). Doing dignity requires an attunement to stratified livability.

In addition to the pressure to earn paychecks, patients' support systems, which might include spouses, long-time partners, family members, church friends, and so on, were also an important part of COVID-19 caretaking. According to participants, patients can benefit immensely from the loving presence of family members, which made limitations on hospital visitation heartbreaking. Patients' kinship networks weren't important just for the patients' own affective support, though. They also supplied HCPs with meaningful background information that could affect the caretaking protocol. When attempting to suss out a dying patient's end-of-life preferences, for example, Luca tactfully asked a series of questions of the patient's adult child via a Zoom call: "What kind of a parent were they? Did they ever ground you?" She continued, "Or my favorite question to ask is, 'What's the craziest thing you've ever lied to your parents about?' There is nothing funnier than seeing a sixty-five-year-old man tell me that they stole beer from their dad back in, you know, 1952 and he still doesn't know about it. And you start to learn about the family dynamic without having to have that conversation with the patient themselves." The need to "learn about the family dynamic" required Luca to be both technologically and rhetorically savvy. But not all patients had charming tales to tell about their family's history. More than once, HCPs brought up the "unsafe discharge."

An unsafe discharge typically indexed when an HCP thought that a patient's caretaking situation after leaving simply was not amenable to survival, let alone recovery. This could be for any number of reasons, but often an unsafe discharge was precipitated by the absence of a supportive home and family environment. In some cases, this absence was related to abuse. But not always. Some patients' caretaking networks simply weren't located in the United States at all, as Kai explained in relating an experience:

> There's one instance that I can think of in my mind of a patient who . . . He was in this field hospital, again non-English-speaking at all. He was from another country, and when he first showed up, he seemed to be getting better. And then after about a week, he started to decline. He wouldn't really talk. His vitals were kind of tanking a little bit. And so we all wondered what was going on. We were going to send them back to the hospital he came from. And one of the team members had suggested, "well, has he had a psych referral?" And we all thought, "psych referral? Why would he need a psych referral?" And so, you know, we asked him if you'd be open to it, and he reluctantly said yes. We sent psych in, and it turns out we had this whole slew of issues related to his family being sick, and there's a lot of violence in the country he had come from, and he was worried about them.

Attuning to patients' often complicated familial histories and kinship networks while also caring for them in a makeshift field hospital in a parking garage meant that the unspoken or misunderstood messaging about a patient's family ties to a war-torn country would be outsourced to psych. COVID-19 patients like Kai's found themselves stuck between here and there, disconnected from the past and anxious about their family's future.

For other patients—and even HCPs themselves—family ties were, sadly, a source of strain during the pandemic. Highlighting childcare constraints, Luca described the toll that remote learning's unpredictability had on her family, who were always living "on a knife's edge." With parents uncertain about whether their children's school would operate in person or remotely, rides to and from medical appointments were disrupted. Grandparents who offered to step in and take care of children were at increased risk of exposure to the virus. And HCPs found themselves caught in the middle. "That's the unfortunate thing," said Idris. "You can identify the fact that, okay, this parent is a single parent that has to go to work, but the kids can't go to daycare because the kid has a cough and so now the parent is in the office, and we have to talk about staying home with the kid and taking care of the kid. And [she] has to make a decision between staying home with the kid or going to work and earning a living. And, I mean, this is a tough conversation we have to have."

Family systems and other kinds of kinship networks have been both a buoy and a burden during the COVID-19 pandemic. Naomi described what was, for me, one of the more shocking examples of how patients' familial backstories—in particular, family guilt—intersected precariously with market-driven medicine. I quote her at length:

> I don't really know how to say this without being accusatory or judgmental . . . [A] situation I run into a lot is patients on hospice being at really nice, really expensive assisted living facilities that charge like ten thousand to twenty thousand dollars a month. And they're really nice. They've got, like cucumbers in their water. They have, I don't know, Zumba aqua therapy, which is great if you are the most vivacious old person in the world with no medical problems. However, assisted living facilities are not medical facilities. The nurses, they're technically not even allowed to give Tylenol or ibuprofen without a script. They can't even technically put Band-Aids on people, legally. So, it's really difficult once you start having a patient who

takes a turn for the worse. And they require a lot more medical care, because the nurses can't facilitate that. There are usually only two or three aides per floor, and hospice only, you know, visits a few times a week . . .

And then you're like, trying to talk to the family about, "Hey, I think we need to get private care because your mom, like she has a pressure ulcer and she's really declining and she's agitated, and you know, based on this facility, it's, it's just not right for her." And families are very resistant to that because they are paying a ton of money just for the rent of being in an assisted living facility. So, they'll say, "No, absolutely not! We're not going to get private care!" And that's, you know, then I scramble as a nurse, because they are in a setting that is not appropriate for their health care needs and . . . sometimes they'll have to end up just like sitting for hours in their own urine. Not necessarily because staff is negligent but because there are two aides for like thirty patients and it just takes time when no one's constantly checking in on them, and so then . . . you know, like they're not getting good care.

And, on the other hand, when you try to say, "well . . . it might not be quite as fancy, but at least I'll get good care," then families tend to get really resistant to that because they don't like the way the environment looks and smells. It definitely feels like an old-person home. We kind of have a saying, colloquially, amongst our colleagues: "The fancier the place is, the bigger the guilt is." You feel like you can just drop off your parents there and just not really be involved because you are paying a huge bill every month.

Familial guilt,[11] coupled with ageism, classism, and capitalism, would exacerbate the friction felt by patients, and HCPs were stuck in the middle. Timely replacement of a urine-soaked bedsheet can hardly be celebrated as dignified care. And yet, a failure to do so would cause a host of undignified asides to fester, wound, and harm.

It probably goes without saying that patients' preexisting conditions, chronic illnesses, and "comorbidities" were also bound up in the sticky caretaking situations described thus far. Chronically ill patients who were scheduled to undergo certain procedures (especially "elective" surgeries) and concomitant follow-up appointments were left hanging. Naomi said, "I have so many clients who are just being dropped for their chronic illness support, and it's really not good. One client lost an eye this fall because she had to have surgery, and they didn't take out her stitches in time. And they got infected, and she lost her eye." Patients weren't the only ones who suffered harms produced at the intersection of preexisting and pandemic conditions. HCPs did as well.

As described earlier, Luca's pre-COVID heart condition put her in the high-risk category according to the Centers of Disease Control and Prevention. But she also spent the early days of the pandemic pregnant. And to top it off, Luca was her mother's primary caregiver: "She's seventy years old and she's immunocompromised. She had breast cancer." Like Idris, Luca found herself internally negotiating feeling perilously prone, suspended among present, past, and future: "So, you know, you don't ever want to skimp on care to a patient, but you also do have to protect yourself and your loved ones." It was hard to begrudge Luca for considering "skimping" on a patient's care when I could hear her breastfeeding her premature newborn daughter as we spoke by phone.

When describing how patients navigated their chronic illnesses and preexisting conditions while recovering from COVID-19, HCPs frequently characterized patients as defeated, depressed, and hopeless. One of Edna's patients had a chronic knee injury compounded by a prolonged COVID-19-related hospital stay: "I don't know what he's doing now, but he had to leave his old job, which was very unfortunate." In this instance, a patient's preexisting condition collided with his current COVID-19 predicament in a way that jeopardized his family's financial future. In such a situation, in/dignities are not isolated to the bedside. They emerge along a continuum of caretaking operations that happen both in and outside the hospital, both before and after acute illness. Doing dignity is "spread out through space and in time" (Mol, 2022, p. 94). There is no "front line." Edna is not a "first responder." The COVID-19 caretaking apparatus does not know boundaries. Doing dignity is a "multiscalar endeavor" that consists of "the little things, and the big things at once" (Fullagar & Pavlidis, 2021, p. 154).

Stuck within such a multiscalar endeavor, Idris found himself participating in what he called a "balancing act" when it came to caring for chronically ill patients. On the one hand, "somebody's A1C might be elevated, but here in this exact moment, I have to prioritize the fact that the goal is to make sure that they can breathe better and they can make it through this illness." When negotiating with a patient, Idris would suggest, "Hey, your sugars are elevated. We got to work on this. But right now, what we're gonna do is we're going to treat your upper respiratory symptoms, and you have to follow up with your care team in two weeks to make sure that your sugars, your diabetic medications are adjusted." Primary care, perpetually prone in time, forces HCPs and their patients to shuttle back and forth between what was, is, and could be. Amplifying such complexity are unaffordable, if not altogether inaccessible, material resources like food, shelter, and transportation. Recognizing the cruelty of asking patients with an elevated A1C to eat healthier when they live in a food desert, Idris confessed, "How are you going to have a low-carb diet when you walk down your street—fast food restaurants all over the place? In the community where I serve, it's considered a low-income community, and so the food choices aren't as healthy . . . [I]t's one thing to talk to them about having a healthy diet, but how do I tell somebody to eat a healthy diet when that means spending more, right?"

A patient having convenient access to healthy food was but one of many infrastructural tubes, lines, and drains frequently clogged, undergoing "routine maintenance," or flat-out unavailable because of buckling global supply chains. Edna referred to these types of contributors to COVID-19 caretaking as "systematic barriers" and saw patients struggle mightily with housing and transportation. About housing, Edna explained,

> People can't pay their rent. The organizations that we usually refer people to where they can get help with their rent are . . . [t]hey are not giving out the money anymore because they're wiped out of funds, and so I think more of the consults are becoming almost like, I don't know how you'd say it, but like people are desperate. They're like, "well let's just call social [work]; they [social work] can figure it out." But things that usually we could help with . . . are so much harder because these resources are hurting, themselves, and don't have the funds and the bandwidth either. So, I think a lot of them have felt like desperation . . . And people are getting angry when you can't, when you're one person, but you can't fix a lot of these problems that have only been [made more] complex with COVID over the last few months, especially as we've gotten further and further

> into this pandemic and people are further and further along with not being able to pay their rent or pay their bills.

On transportation, Edna told us,

> I had a lot of dialysis patients who obviously were living in a crowded area, crowded apartments with multiple people or homeless, and they were getting COVID but still needed to do dialysis. And the biggest struggle I had was people getting appropriate transportation. They would use the bus or the train, living, you know, where I live—in an urban area. And they couldn't do that anymore. There were all these restrictions with the dialysis centers, saying they can't take a cab because you're putting that person at risk, and they have to know that they're transporting someone who has COVID-19.

All participants recognized the value of telehealth services given how complex transportation had become for many patients like Edna's. As with most things, though, for every affordance one solution offered, a host of adjacent constraints emerged in a ripple effect, especially when insurance companies' policies were out of sync with current pandemic conditions. In the early days of the pandemic, some patients' insurance companies were unwilling to pay for telehealth; what's more, some patients simply didn't have access to the technology required for telehealth, as Idris explained:

> There are people that live in communities in [redacted] where they can't get on a computer if they wanted to. Now, in the old days, they would go to the library or to a medical facility and be hooked on. But you can't just all of a sudden show up at the library and be put on a computer and talk to your doctor. So, I think that's going to add a new dimension to disparity of how we, if we are going to expand things like telehealth, how we're going to do it so patients can afford to do it.

Other undignified asides were less materially tangible during COVID-19 caretaking but still had a pernicious presence—including, and especially, both implicit and explicit biases.[12] Gendered, racialized, ableist, classist, and political biases were formidable factors for COVID-19 caretakers. Luca frequently found herself caring for "older . . . extremely independent and self-reliant" men who "don't ever want to be a bother" or to "admit that there's anything wrong or that they need anything." Over time, Luca described developing a heightened attunement to patients who, even when struggling to breathe, were hamstrung by gender-based expectations for how to behave:

> He was probably about in his eighties, and he was a hardworking man all his life and had been fairly healthy, and then . . . he got COVID and then was transferred to our floor and was just really having a hard time adjusting [to] being on six liters of oxygen, taking a bunch of medication. And so, he was having some pain in his chest, and he didn't want to say anything because he didn't want to be a bother. So, I can kind of pick up on the nonverbal cues and his mannerisms and his face. And then the more time that you spend with patients, the more you get to know them and know when things aren't right.

Other HCPs, like Kai, described how political biases seeded several un/dignified asides. After having spent some of the earliest days of the pandemic in Italy, where he attended medical school, Kai found himself making comparisons between how the United States and Italy enacted "solidarity":

> Yeah, I think solidarity is a good way to put it. Everyone there [in Italy] wears masks. They [Italians] don't really question science or the government. Unfortunately, America, I mean, America is obviously a very multicultural place, a great country; yet, it's very hard for every citizen to agree on one thing, and I think, unfortunately, that contributed to COVID; just, you know, it just kept getting worse here. I mean, there were the anti-maskers, and obviously we had lots of social protest, which weren't ideal, but . . . I don't know. In Italy, it's a smaller country. It's really difficult to compare the two countries, but I think they just had more solidarity. They were more scared of the virus . . . Italians, they took it pretty seriously. Some people, you know, would not go to bars. Here, I have friends that are just kind of like, you know, "if I get the virus, I get the virus." So, I think the whole attitude to the virus there is a little different. They're a smaller country, again, with an aging population, and they took it more seriously.

Kai also had to discover how to provide care to patients who say "really racist stuff":

> And you're just like holy, like . . . All right, I didn't know we were going down that road. I really don't want to talk about that with you. I have extremely different views on this than you. But even though all of that is true, it doesn't change the underlying fact, which is I'm here to be a provider for you, and you have real needs. And because of that I should do everything within my power to prevent anything from disrupting that care because that's, that's my mission.

This was but one of many examples in which an HCP from an underrepresented community was forced to care for someone who despised them.

Avoiding care disruptions, despite harmful ideologies, was made more difficult when the approach to care itself was politicized. Luca, for example, contended not just with anti-maskers but also with families who had clearly been affected by dominant discourses around the "war on drugs":

> It could come off as offensive. Like, "how dare you say you're going to drug up my mom!" Or, "how dare you say you're going to sedate my dad, where he can't interact with us anymore!" And so, it definitely is a gray area where you could be offending somebody, and it could come off as undignified care very easily. And, you know, obviously we do everything in our power to avoid scenarios like that, but it definitely happens. I think it's more common, those gray areas, than people think. And that is simply because every patient is different. Doesn't matter how many years I've worked . . . how much experience our team has. Every single patient is different, and that makes gray areas, very, very common.

So-called gray areas resulting from clashing beliefs were abundant. More than a single individual's belief system or political conviction, though, said biases were often the product of larger forces and failures rendered invisible by health care policies and procedures. Luca described a situation where a 43-year-old COVID-19 patient with no prior health issues needed a double lung transplant: "Unfortunately, she was an illegal immigrant, so they're obviously not going to jump on getting her that because she has no insurance or anything." Even now as I type that, I remain struck by the fact that Luca saw a delayed double lung transplant as the "obvious" outcome for "an illegal immigrant," especially since she acknowledged that "she was almost looked at differently" or "looked down on . . . because she was here illegally." Luca's acquiescence to what resulted at the intersection of ethnonationalism and a global health crisis demonstrates how the US caretaking apparatus continues to function based on harmful biopolitical assumptions about certain humans' un/worthiness. In plain sight is what Weheliye (2014) describes as a "discourse of putative scarcity" wherein patients like Luca's "compete for limited resources" (p. 14); what results is not just this patient's likely death but also "a strengthening of the very mechanisms that deem certain groups more disposable or not-quite-human than others" (p. 14).

Adjacent to anti-immigration biases were ableist logics, both of which were most certainly amplified by the US president at the time of this study. Troubled by all the patients who "fall through the cracks," Naomi told us about one client in particular:

> [He] lives alone, has Parkinson's. Can't cook. Doesn't have any family. Has no car . . . Just really isolated. Lives in a tiny dark, dark room. Doesn't ever turn on the lights. Doesn't ever open the blinds. Never goes out. Skinny, tiny, like, really super depressed. And he never, he didn't have services. And I, I started delivering Meals on Wheels to him, and I was like . . . I realized he's . . . someone that I could get on services, so I referred him to start getting personal care. And I trained the worker to go with him. And like, it just it was like, "Thank God." You know, I mean, it, it's . . . made such a difference to have someone that goes in there every day and just helps him make lunch, you know?

When I followed up with Naomi to inquire about how this client was faring now that he'd been given access to personal care services, she replied,

> Oh, yeah. Yeah. I mean, he's . . . [h]e talks, he smiles. He goes out with her for walks. Like he has a little scooter, and he wasn't able to get it out because his apartment isn't accessible. He can't drive the scooter out of his apartment at the same time as holding the door open. I mean, it's just, you know, these stupid things, you know, that are barriers. So, she takes him out on the scooter, and he gets out some fresh air. And he wasn't able to do that before.

If nothing else, one of the major findings from this project is how significant social workers and home health aides are for finding ways to intercede on behalf of clients who, as Naomi described, "fall through the cracks." Constant exposure to others' exposedness, however, took a toll on HCPs like Naomi. After describing how many of her clients' hoarding behaviors increased during COVID-19, she noted that she's always "trying to find a way to help a home-care worker work effectively in those environments, without being judgmental. Without being, like, critical or disgusted, you know, let's just say it. Like, it's hard . . . It can really transform someone."

A consistent theme among all the HCPs was burnout, especially when we asked about the impact COVID-19 had on mental health. When participants were asked about a time they may have witnessed or experienced "undignified care" during the pandemic, anyone who had a story to tell seemed to blame it on burnout, such as Naomi's: "It would be them, or anybody on the team, not checking in with themselves and not realizing they're burnt out . . . I feel often that they need more than we're able to give. And we don't have the volunteers anymore, and you don't have the family members, and it's just, you know, you try to be more than adequate but sometimes it's . . . I feel just overwhelmed." In addition to feeling overwhelmed, Kai described burnout as accompanied by "a little bit of nihilism that creeps in." Kai's colleagues who worked in an infectious disease ward "were absolutely overwhelmed come March, April, and May. Yeah, they were working overtime. Many of them got the virus . . . One in the department unfortunately died . . . PPE was obviously [in short supply] . . . We were running out of resources." Naomi, indeed all the HCPs in this study, had to grapple with the ways "an invisible non-living agent" became "alive in bodies and halted the flow of capital, people and commodities, causing global supply chains" to falter (Fullagar & Pavlidis, 2021, p. 155).

Uncertainty caused by global supply chain failures resulted in resource rationing. Naomi was furious about how "underfunded and understaffed" her agency was. The home health workers she supervised were, in her words, horribly exploited: "I mean, they're not given enough PPE to begin with, and it's rationed. It's been rationed since the beginning, and we still don't have any N-95s right now." In response to Naomi's indignation, critical health researchers might draw attention to the role of union busting, which targets "labor unions with the goal of minimizing their bargaining rights if not completely eliminating them" (Dutta, 2016, p. 28). At the same time, most of the clients that Naomi's agency was responsible for were "totally dependent on the state-based benefits programs . . . [T]hey are extremely poor. Significant disability. Often, they're living in public housing, with vouchers from the state. All of their medical care is through Medicaid." Weary from the ways COVID-19 care was prone between union busting, or "biopolitical regulation," and "state recognition of vulnerability" (Oliviero, p. 248), Naomi's voice cracked when she told us, "So, you know, getting them what they need is really hard."

Describing how "the system" employed "algorithms of need" when determining how to ration care, Naomi told us another astonishing story about a patient who went to bed at five o'clock in the afternoon—not by choice but because a host of intersecting structural indignities can make home health care in the United States a horrifying experience.

> So, for example, I have a client, who's quadriplegic. Lives alone in public housing, and in [redacted], where I live, there's a PCA [personal care attendant] program. I don't know if it's in other states, similarly, but it's very different than a health aid program. It's an independent-living model, where the consumer—*they're called consumers*—are the employer, and they hire and fire and train their personal care attendants. And they manage them. Much like an employer, except the relationship is really unique between the worker and the consumer. Usually, it's much more casual, much more non-professionalized. I tend to prefer that relationship to the one . . . that I work within, which is much more about hired services. And, so, there's often this conflict: The state authorizes a certain number of hours that someone is qualified for. And usually, it's never enough. And so the person—*the consumer*—has to ration their hours and make bargains with their PCAs and make incentives for their PCAs. And, you know, in order to just get what they need to be able to get up in the morning and get a shower, or have a meal at dinnertime or go to bed at, you know . . .
>
> I have one client who goes to bed at five o'clock, because he doesn't have someone available, when he would prefer to go to bed at nine o'clock

> or ten o'clock . . . Or, his wheelchair has been broken for like two weeks, and he can't get out of bed without his wheelchair. So, now he's in bed for two weeks. Is that dignified? No. Is that honoring his wishes to be able to have a productive and active life? No . . . And because of these, you know, bureaucratic programs, no one is really, ultimately held responsible.

Built into the home health care model Naomi describes is an "analogy between health behaviors and products or services. Health is understood as an individual choice presented within a marketplace" (Dutta, 2016, p. 27). Clearly, there are only a certain number of choices available within market-based models for care. Being forced to go to bed at five o'clock hardly lends support for such a model. We heard a similar story of the US health care system's reliance on market-driven "algorithms of need" when Idris described how he and his colleagues had to spend one after-hours shift combing through patient charts to decide who could survive being prematurely removed from their feeding tube. Due to a national shortage in feeding tube pumps, Idris and his team were responsible for determining who could survive premature feeding tube removal in order to sustain another patient who needed a feeding tube to survive.

Suspended *In Medias Res*

> But those people who are being proned, they don't like it. They turn themselves back onto their back. They then desaturate their oxygen levels, and then it's just a constant battle, trying to reiterate, you need to do this, you need to do that.
>
> —*Focus Group Participant, 12/14/2020*

In the next chapter about death-with-dignity legislation, I describe how some persons wish to hasten their death because they feel as though they're a burden—a burden to their families, loved ones, and the larger US health care apparatus. But such a sentiment is not expressed only in conversations about end-of-life legislation. Some HCPs in this study said that, even among patients who weren't at the end of their lives, some asked for suicide assistance. "They told me they feel [like] a burden,"

Naomi recounted. "They don't like to have someone doing their personal care. It's embarrassing . . . The system doesn't provide for people. And rather than fighting the system to get what people need, they actually are opting to die. *They would rather die.* And to me, that's frightening. Because it's almost like this hopelessness about an inability to change the world for a better place, you know." As Mbembe (2019) describes, "nearly everywhere the political order is reconstituting itself as a form of organization for death" (p. 7). I have hours of interview and focus group data that point to how COVID-19 care was a fraught, necropolitical enterprise, not just because of factors at the bedside but also because of a host of infrastructural failures and market-driven forces. Is it any wonder, then, that some patients expressed hopelessness?

Unaddressed thus far is the fact that, as Naomi described, "most people I know . . . have experienced harm from the medical system." This, too, was a part of COVID-19 caretaking's infrastructural inheritance. Indeed, the US health care system's legacy is made up of decades of medical harm perpetrated on disabled people and on Black, Indigenous, and other people of color (cf. Harriet A. Washington's [2006] *Medical Apartheid*). Persons who have experienced such harm employed various tactics for taking care while receiving care during the pandemic. Kai, for example, described how some patients created alliances with their roommates: "All the sudden, Jim from PT [physical therapy] is just like the worst person ever because . . . unclear to me maybe what Jim did, but . . . Jim worked with patient A in that room, Susie, and then you know went to work with Jolene, Susie's roommate the next day, and [she] was like 'oh hell no, you're the worst!' " Alliances emerged on all sides of the caretaking apparatus, though. For example, after caring for an incarcerated patient, Luca described how, afterwards, a prison guard pulled her aside and said, "you know, he molested his little sister." While Luca was adamant that such information would not cause her to discriminate against a patient, Kai described a senior colleague who had a reputation for unabashedly documenting his discrimination: "There is a nephrologist who writes really horrific things in patients' charts . . . [H]e'll write like, 'maybe patient should consider stop being a rapist in order to improve his kidney function.' It's like, oh my God. I mean, you can't write that." Importantly, Kai seemed to recognize that what was documented in a pa-

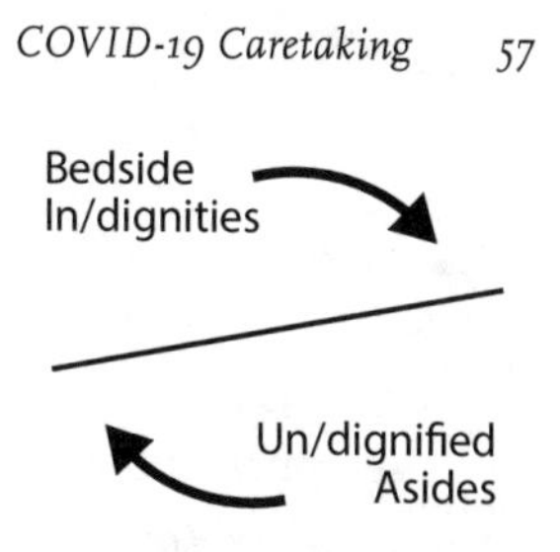

Figure 2.2. COVID-19 caretaking straddles domains, including both bedside in/dignities and un/dignified asides.

tient's chart would become a part of that patient's caretaking inheritance going forward. Numerous HCPs did, indeed, express trepidation about entering a new patient's room because of something a colleague had written about them in their chart.

Narratives from Edna, Luca, Kai, Idris, and Naomi illustrate how fraught COVID-19 caretaking—and caretaking, in general—is, with its host of local and larger in/dignities that seed and feed on one another. As such, "*doing good* becomes a task to take on stubbornly, even if—or precisely because—it is tantalizingly elusive" (Mol, 2021, p. 100). As Alaimo (2016) and many other material feminists and critical posthumanists have argued, "the domains of the ethical and the political, the personal and the public, the domestic and the global, have collapsed into each other" (p. 10). Although a still image cannot capture collapse happening over time, the off-kilter line crossing figure 2.2 attempts to illustrate just that. This tidy visual falls short of representing caretaking's complexity, even though it helps me close the existential pronation loop with which this chapter began. "Suspended within complex normative force fields," Mol (2021) tells us, "*doing* goes on and on. It never comes to rest" (p. 143). Indeed, COVID-19 caretaking is more of a necropolitical *mangle*—a mangle of bedside in/dignities and un/dignified asides—than a balanced, closed system as figure 2.2 would suggest (see Pickering, 1993).

As a disorienting mangle of material-discursive phenomena, COVID-19 caretaking is perpetually suspended between here and there, this and that, you and me. And so, we try to corral the chaos through policies and procedures, but the knottiness persists. The mangle of bedside in/dignities and un/dignified asides are, as Arendt (1958/2013) might say, "the story that an act starts"; in other words, the in/actions described throughout this chapter occur in "a medium where every reaction becomes a chain reaction and where every process is the cause of a new process" (p. 190). Attempting to "offer realistic hope," in Kai's words, HCPs were constantly looking for ways to navigate a space between desensitized nihilism and the kind of naïve sentimentality described in the opening of chapter one. They were weary, Kai admitted: "It's just, it's hard to keep hope in those situations where you have someone who's in a high-risk group, comorbid conditions, or old age, whatever it may be. And you have nothing to give them. You just have to say, you have this virus. It can be very fatal in some instances, and we just need to keep close monitoring you. It's not very reassuring for myself or for the patient. That's probably the biggest challenge right now."

In place of "realistic hope," Idris offered honesty: "They don't know whether or not their infection is going to lead to their mortality . . . And so, I have these conversations with people, and I'm really honest with them." Given the infrastructural forces and failures with which patients, clients, and HCPs alike must contend, it's clear that COVID-19 caretaking is more of "a political condition" than an "individualized experience" (Oliviero, 2018, p. 26). At one time or another, each element of the caretaking apparatus is prone between the local and political as well as the individual and institutional.

The potential for in/dignity is always caught between. It's in the postures and poses that go unnamed. It's in the gestures expressed on the way toward a point—it's in "passage rather than position" (Yergeau, 2018, p. 66). In/dignities emerge in slivers of un/accompanied abiding and abandonment. Within the COVID-19 caretaking apparatus, in other words, in/dignities hover *in medias res*. Dignity never fully settles in. Suspended in both time and space, un/dignified care happens in the interstices of COVID caretaking, the material-discursive emplacements betwixt the immediacy of the bedside and all that's come before and will come after. More present than ever are the otherwise unseen forces that many privileged persons at another time might well ignore. This chapter illustrates how care is what happens on the way from and toward what Hulme and Truch (2005) call "interspaces." Like proning, in/dignities at the bedside and beyond turn things around.

Caretaking requires, at the very least, a sensitivity (if not responsivity) to a host of inheritances—all of which accrete over time to condition stratified livability. Each "composite narrative" (Saldaña & Omasta, 2022; Willis, 2019) described in this chapter highlights the many ways that HCPs engaged in "conflict-solving dignity work" (Örulv & Nikku, 2007, p. 510) during the COVID-19 pandemic. By reseeing in/dignity as perpetually suspended *in medias res*—acting on and acted upon by a host of local conditions and larger conditionalities—un/dignified care might be seen as a series of coterminous, wearying experiences and tasks that accrue over time and in space.[13] As Naomi remarked when asked about human dignity, "It's a process . . . a relationship . . . It's not about something that you inherently have. It's about something that is created *between* . . . Between!" In the next two case studies, readers will witness some of the backstage logics and preconditions that fortify such in-between spaces.

CHAPTER THREE

Death-with-Dignity's Biopolitical Topoi

> . . . choice is illusory in a context of pervasive inequality. Choices are structured by oppression. We shouldn't offer assistance with suicide until we all have the assistance we need to get out of bed in the morning and live a good life.
>
> —*Harriet McBryde Johnson, "Unspeakable Conversations"*

For advocates of the right to choose when and how to end your life, or what some call "death-with-dignity," 2019 was the most successful legislative year ever. Proponents of death-with-dignity legislation, more recently referred to as "medical aid in dying" (MAiD), noted that "for the first time, two states—Maine and New Jersey—passed assisted-dying laws in the same year. Simultaneously, 18 additional state legislatures considered physician-assisted death bills, some for the first time" (DeathWithDignity.org, n.d.). At the same time that hearings on MAiD legislation have increased in the United States, the suicide rate has never been higher. And, as I write this, the United States has just surpassed one million COVID-19-related deaths. It may seem incongruous that while state legislatures are trying to *prevent* people from dying, they are also deliberating about how to *hasten* death legally for people with so-called life-limiting conditions.

These are not the only incongruities that have emerged around MAiD deliberations in the United States.[1] One critic of MAiD recently testified that the matter of legislating who and how one can die "doesn't fit at all into traditional red and blue [political] categories":

> You have progressives testifying before this committee sounding like libertarians, arguing on the basis of individual freedom, autonomy, and government staying away from the choices of the individual. Meanwhile, you have conservatives sounding like left-wing activists: talking about nonviolence, showing true care and concern for the most vulnerable, and doing analysis of the unintended structural evils that are created when physician-assisted suicide is legalized. Most bizarrely of all, you have the party of business and wealth doing an implicit critique of capitalism—by insisting that one's value does not come from autonomy, productivity, or how much you "contribute to society." But rather simply because of the fundamental equality of all.[2]

MAiD testimony such as the one cited above exemplifies the paradox I described in chapter one: when it comes to matters of human dignity, warrants mobilized by interlocutors on opposite sides of a biopolitical controversy occasionally and surprisingly share common rhetorical ground. To examine how various incongruities and paradoxes develop during deliberations about death and dying, this chapter reports results from my rhetorical analyses of contemporary death-with-dignity discourse that participants employed during public hearings about MAiD legislation. For this case study, I analyzed death-with-dignity discourse in US legislative debates at the state level—specifically, debates about whether, when, and how certain residents should receive legally sanctioned assistance from a medical provider to hasten their own death.

One of the strongest advocates of death-with-dignity legislation is the Compassion & Choices Action Network, a nonprofit organization located in Portland, Oregon, that has an impressive presence all around the United States. The cornerstone of its campaign is that death-with-dignity is *not* assisted suicide. Rather, according to Compassion & Choices' website, MAiD legislation improves care, expands options, and empowers dying persons and their families (compassionandchoices.org). One of the reasons MAiD proponents from Compassion & Choices and a related organization, Death with Dignity, are pleased with the increase in legis-

TABLE 3.1.
MAiD legislation in 10 US states and the District of Columbia

Statute	State	Year in effect
Death with Dignity Act	Oregon	1994 (stayed), 1997
Death with Dignity Act	Washington	2008
No statute in place; state supreme court ruled that nothing in state's laws prohibited physician-assisted dying	Montana	2009
Patient Choice and Control at End-of-Life Act	Vermont	2013
End of Life Options Act	California	2015
End of Life Options Act	Colorado	2016
Death with Dignity Act	District of Columbia	2017
Our Care, Our Choice Act	Hawaii	2018
Death with Dignity Act	Maine	2019
Aid in Dying for the Terminally Ill Act	New Jersey	2019
End of Life Options Act	New Mexico	2021

lative action regarding MAiD is because, at the time I write this, only 10 US states and the District of Columbia have successfully enacted some form of MAiD legislation (table 3.1).[3]

Note that no names of MAiD laws in table 3.1. contain phrases such as "assisted suicide" or "euthanasia." Moreover, the "physician" (once centered in "physician-assisted suicide") has been replaced by depersonalized "medical" aid in dying. These discursive shifts signal how governing bodies are changing the terms by which we describe, debate, and practice dignity at the end of life. MAiD proponents are attempting to rebrand the practice in ways that, at least discursively, distance themselves from accusations that they are promoting suicide or euthanasia.

It may be tempting to think that MAiD proponents' rebranding efforts are attempts at political correctness. However, more than five decades ago—long before the trope of political correctness emerged—the US Senate's Special Committee on Aging held a death-with-dignity legislative hearing that highlighted the importance of word choice. During the hearing's introductory remarks, Chairperson Frank Church admonished his colleagues: "This inquiry is not a hearing on euthanasia . . . [T]here is a great difference between what he and others envision as 'death-with-dignity' and what others call 'mercy deaths.' Let me emphasize again that this hearing has nothing to do with euthanasia" (*Death with dignity*, 1972, p. 1). Politicians have always been concerned with the words used to describe the legislative enactment of death-with-dignity.

Inspired by shifting discourse around death-with-dignity, this chapter builds on critical health research that investigates "how bodies are governed by discourses of health and wellness" (Pringle, 2019, p. 1). The fundamental assumption guiding this chapter is that legislative acts governing who, how, or when someone dies are, themselves, powerful forms of biopolitical discourse that condition stratified livability. Introduced in chapter one, stratified livability as a construct indexes the effects of "socio-economic inequalities, racial discrimination and uneven access to healthcare" (Manderson, Burke, & Wahlberg, 2021, p. 2) and highlights how "some will—and some must—die in order that others may live" (Murray, p. 24).

As I have already identified, words that index MAiD legislation are under constant scrutiny. But because public policymaking involves "mediating rhetorical and material elements" (Asen, 2010, p. 129), passing MAiD legislation requires an attunement to states' local material conditions, as well. For example, often embedded in MAiD testimony are residents' religious convictions, socioeconomic constraints, assumptions about what it is like to live with a disability, and even adjacent public health debates about who is responsible for rising rates of teen suicide or the overuse of prescription painkillers. Such factors contribute to what the previous chapter termed "un/dignified asides." I argue that when harmful biopolitical logics take center stage during public policy hearings about MAiD legislation, un/dignified asides become normalized. One way to interrupt the normalization of un/dignified asides is to name them. That is my goal for this chapter.

By untangling the argumentative premises—or what I call biopolitical *topoi* (singular: *topos*)—that structure un/dignified care at the end of life, this chapter details how contemporary death-with-dignity discourse frames some persons as more biopolitically disposable than others. I hope that by identifying and discussing MAiD deliberations' biopolitical topoi, readers will reflect on the ways we might be complicit in normalizing logics of care/lessness. Rosemarie Garland-Thompson (2017a) might refer to such normalizing logics as a type of "eugenic world building"—a construct that she employs when critiquing the commonplace ableism in Kazuo Ishiguro's *Never Let Me Go*. Eugenic world building, according to Garland-Thompson, "strives to eliminate disability and, along with it, people with disabilities from human communities and future worlds through varying social and material practices that range from seemingly benign to egregiously unethical" (n.p.). For the purposes of this chapter, I'm interested in uncovering how MAiD deliberators' biopolitical topoi (however "seemingly benign") normalize indignity.

Michael Hyde (2006) describes topoi as " 'places'—issues, values, commitments, beliefs, likelihoods—that we hold in common with others, that we *dwell in* and *argue over*, and that we use reflectively to find the issues and premises of a specific case" (p. 70; emphasis in the original). During MAiD testimony, topoi emerge from "a repertoire of responses to practical problems that the thoughtful inquirer can turn to for *re*-sources—sources that can be used again and again on opposite sides of a question as new problems occur" (Hyde, p. 70). Results from my rhetorical analysis of biopolitical topoi in MAiD testimony unveil the "moral predicates" that underpin how human dignity is governed at the end of life (Zemlicka, 2013, p. 276). Furthermore, my analysis shows how dignity rarely stands on its own. Rather, dignity is often tethered to (or hijacked by) sentimentalized ableism, among other logics of care/lessness. What emerges, then, is a dominant discourse about death-with-dignity that hinges on the pathologizing of dependency.

Pathologized dependency tends to hide out in universalizing assertions about compassion and choice. Recall from chapter one the litany of scholars who critique "the universalist pretentions of Western humanism" (Mbembe, 2019, p. 161). Such critiques became especially apt after I spent time with testimony that echoed Compassion & Choices' pro-MAiD arguments. Yoked to universalizing assertions about human compassion and individual choice were MAiD interlocutors' ableist assumptions about toileting, "life in a wheelchair," being a burden, and the need to ration care to those who stand to benefit the most from it. How everyday persons talk about options for death and dying sheds light on prevailing logics of care/lessness—logics that, when scaled up to policy, condition some persons as more biopolitically disposable than others. Revealing and redressing such dominant discourses is necessary for reimagining the "new genre" of human dignity described in chapter one (Wynter, 2003).

To understand how logics of care/lessness underwrite certain persons' biopolitical disposability, I have sacrificed representativeness or generalizability in exchange for depth and detail by delimiting the scope of my analysis to five public hearings regarding MAiD in Nevada and Connecticut. I report results from rhetorical analyses of how arguments for or against MAiD legislation unfolded in these two states. Why Nevada and Connecticut? Coincidence and convenience. Hearings in these two states were taking place as I was drafting a chapter on what would be an analysis of how extant death-with-dignity legislation framed dignity discursively. One afternoon, while I was reading existing MAiD legislation, I received a Google alert informing me that the State of Connecticut was holding a hearing on proposed MAiD legislation. Because of COVID-19, the hearing was held over Zoom and livestreamed on YouTube. So, I tuned in. Parts of the hearing were mere bureaucratic processes, but other parts were riveting.

I was bowled over, in fact, by more than 10 hours of testimony from Connecticut residents and representatives from relevant nonprofit organizations. After the hearing concluded, I abandoned my original plan to analyze texts proposing MAiD legislation and chose instead to analyze public deliberations about said legislation. In addition to listening to digital recordings of hearings (where available), I also examined written minutes from hearings and accessible written testimony and proposed amendments. The Connecticut corpus includes written and verbal testimony from two legislative hearings about MAiD in 2021 and 2022. The Nevada corpus includes written testimony from three different legislative hearings about MAiD in 2017, 2019, and 2021.

Scholars in health communication and medical rhetoric have for some time studied the complexity of end-of-life decision making (e.g., Barton, 2007; Keränen, 2007; McDorman, 2005; Schryer et al., 2012; Schuster et al. 2013, 2014; Segal, 2000a); this chapter adds to that literature by taxonomizing the material-discursive logics of care/lessness that structure, if not predetermine, end-of-life options in the first place. In other words, locally situated logics of care/lessness have consequences for if and how one may choose to die in Nevada and Connecticut. And these consequences are not evenly distributed. Some persons experience more of an infrastructural burden when navigating dignified life and death, while other persons may in fact feel empowered to control what dignity looks like for them. This, too, exemplifies what I described in chapter one as stratified livability.

Michael Hyde (2001b) notes that controversies such as MAiD could be "decided by those who end up telling the best stories" (p. 178). And, indeed, that appears to be the case; consider what Senator Will Haskell of Connecticut shared in a post-hearing press release:

> The stories I've heard will keep me up at night. With courageous candor, my constituents have shared what it is like to be forced to live with the knowledge of their impending deaths, and also the crushing physical and emotional pain of that final chapter," said Sen. Haskell. "I've decided to co-sponsor this legislation, because I believe these patients should have the right to live their final days in a manner of their choosing. In looking to other states, we know that this can be done in a way that promotes safety, autonomy, and dignity for all. ("I don't want," 2021)

Senator Haskell's supportive stance on MAiD, as evidenced by his decision to cosponsor Connecticut's bill, is backed up by certain biopolitical topoi, or rhetorical commonplaces, on which interlocutors hinge their stance on a (necropolitically) fraught matter. Uncovering biopolitical topoi is one mechanism for tracing the logics of care/lessness that support an individual's MAiD stance.

It isn't just the "good stories" that compel me to analyze MAiD testimony's biopolitical topoi. I am also motivated by the fact that numerous paradigm shifts in death-with-dignity discourse are unaccounted for in extant scholarship. Nearly two decades ago, Margaret Pabst Battin (2005) identified five "principal arguments" in the MAiD debate, which at the time was called "physician-assisted suicide," or PAS (table 3.2). Battin's pathbreaking "paradigmatic argument-scheme about physician-assisted suicide" makes the case that "there are two mainstay issues in the 'pro'-PAS column: the autonomy argument" and the compassionate "relief of pain and suffering" argument (p. 406). Battin's work certainly broke new ground at the time, but much has changed since 2005, especially in the United States.

TABLE 3.2.
Battin's (2005) argumentative schema among MAiD supporters versus opponents

Principal arguments *for* MAiD	Principal arguments *against* MAiD
Argument from autonomy Argument from relief of pain and suffering	Argument from intrinsic wrongness of killing Argument from professional integrity Argument from potential abuse of law if passed; beware the slippery slope

Implicit in Battin's first principles is the assumption that one's religious convictions or political party affiliation probably map on to their stance on MAiD. (For instance, whereas Democrats prioritize bodily autonomy, the religious Right prioritizes God's commandment "Thou shall not kill.") But recall the testimony with which I opened this chapter. Today, one's stance on MAiD tends not to correlate neatly with a person's religious or political beliefs. Certainly, popular discourse about US politics suggests that US voters are more polarized than ever; but when it comes to biopolitical controversies such as MAiD, the lines are somewhat blurred among residents (though not necessarily among politicians, who still, by and large, back or oppose MAiD legislation along party lines). To be sure, many MAiD opponents continue to mobilize religious belief as an argumentative warrant. But I posit that the dismissive rebuttal that all MAiD opponents are religious zealots who disrespect the separation of church and state is both reductive and less rhetorically effective than it once was.

Second, in response to Battin's and copious others' examinations of the "slippery slope" premise, contemporary MAiD legislators (including those in Nevada and Connecticut) have amended their bills to incorporate dozens of "safeguards" that are designed to act as legal guardrails against sliding down a slippery slope. Among numerous other safeguards are a host of "eligibility conditions," for example. That is, to be eligible for MAiD, one must be at least 18 years of age, possess "decision-making capacity," and be "terminally ill." These safeguards have provoked definitional questions, such as how is someone's "decision-making capacity" to be determined,[4] or how do physicians determine "terminal status" (Barton, 2005, p. 261)? But I argue that what remains of the slippery-slope objection is complex enough to justify its parsing, rather than dismissively lumping all slippery-slope appeals into a single logical fallacy.

Third, echoing Battin, several scholars have pointed out how death-with-dignity discourse is warranted by cultural conventions for how people characterize a "good death"—specifically, the degree to which pain and suffering is or ought to be a natural part of dying.[5] While such arguments are not necessarily moot, it's worth noting that increased access to palliative care, hospice, and advanced directives have lessened the argumentative strength of such premises.[6] Moreover, scholars attuned to medicalized racism rightly point out how "good death" discussions tend to be "grounded in a privileged standpoint that centers the concerns of white educated persons" (Jennings & Talley, 2003). Definitions of a "good death," then, are rooted in racialized assemblages (Weheliye, 2014), which Battin's schema overlooks.

Finally, the politicization of the Affordable Care Act (cf. the racialization of Obamacare's "death panels") paired with COVID-19's disruption of the global supply chain described in chapter two made palpable previously dismissed paranoia about resource rationing in health care. As readers will witness, a good deal of contemporary discourse about MAiD hinges on concerns about the unsustainable cost of health care and the role of insurance companies in reifying the racializing assemblages responsible for pervasive health disparities. Embedded in the tension between affordability and access is a legitimate skepticism about whether, by making MAiD legal, insurance companies will advocate for assisted dying instead of footing the bill for costly medical treatments. Furthermore, in states where MAiD is legal, those who choose to use such legislation are overwhelmingly and disproportionately white and upper/middle class. End-of-life care in the United States, more broadly, is already listed as one of many health disparities (see, for example, Ornstein et al., 2020).

Said simply, the matter of death-with-dignity is complex enough that it is worth revisiting how everyday people reason about and evidentially support their stance on MAiD. In his article "Vernacular Discourse and the Epistemic Dimension of Public Opinion," Gerard Hauser (2007) encourages readers to pay greater attention to "exchanges among ordinary citizens that underwrite public opinion" (p. 333), especially given "the Internet's power to form public opinion and communicate it to decision makers in ways that are consequential" (p. 338). Hauser distinguishes between public opinion polls, expert voices, and what he calls "reasoned dialogue among actively engaged citizens who are making and tending to arguments on an issue" (p. 334). For Hauser, "media moguls" (p. 339) and the surveys that quantify current trends in public opinion about complex matters (such as MAiD) may not account for the richness of firsthand experiences that citizens describe via what he calls vernacular discourse. Citizens' personal narratives enable researchers to understand people's "depth of conviction" (p. 334) on a matter. To that I would add that personal narratives allow us to see how intersecting material concerns—un/dignified asides—shape citizens' stances on complex matters such as MAiD. Accounting for these concerns might also shed light on why MAiD is disproportionately used by wealthy white people. Because the words "citizen" and "citizenship" are fraught with biopolitical complexity, I use "interlocutor" to refer to someone who testified on MAiD or, when applicable, "resident" or "representative" of a state or organization.

Rhetoricians investigate vernacular discourses in order to understand "norms of reasoning, standards of evidence, and modes of argumentation" that may not necessarily align with the norms, evidential standards, and argumentative modes employed by "politicians, political parties, and power elites" (Hauser, 2007, pp. 339, 337). My sense is that a widespread assumption about MAiD deliberations in this contemporary moment is that most Left-leaning, liberal humanists support death-with-dignity, while only outdated logics about religion and morality substantiate the position of MAiD opponents. My analyses reveal, however, that MAiD legislation, despite multiple efforts at rebranding, is not only "deblackened and unraced" (Douglass, 2018, p. 106) but is also reliant on "eugenic logics" (Garland-Thompson, 2017a) that pathologize dependency. MAiD legislation and the dominant discourses that circulate around it proffer a universalized notion of the human (cf. Jackson, 2020) that privileges compulsory able-bodiedness (McRuer, 2010).

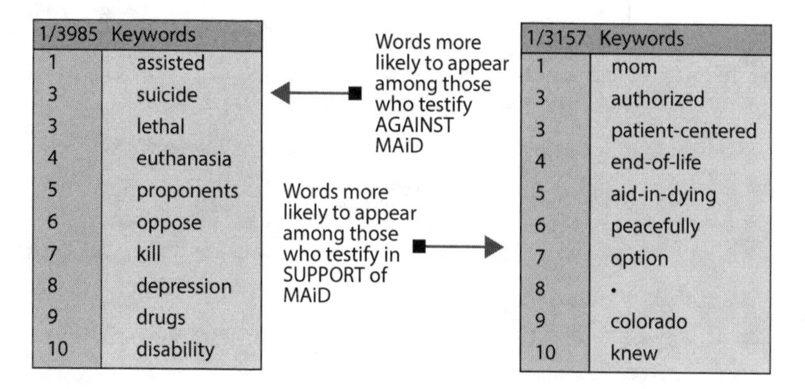

Figure 3.1. Results of LancsBox's corpus analysis of MAiD testimony. Words that were more likely to be used by those who testified against MAiD are in the *left* column; words more likely to be used by those who testified in support of MAiD are in the *right* column. (Disregard the bullet.)

First Analytic Approach: Corpus Linguistics

To generate an initial impression of potential correlations between interlocutors' discourse and their stance on MAiD, I mobilized tools from corpus linguistics. One corpus linguistic software program, LancsBox (Brezina, Weill-Tessier, & McEnery, 2020), renders visual representations of "collocation graphs and networks . . . to show associations and cross-associations between words in language and discourse" (Brezina, 2018). Two lists in figure 3.1 show which words were most frequently used by MAiD opponents and which words were most frequently used by MAiD proponents.

LancsBox compared words from two corpora that I, along with two research assistants,[7] painstakingly assembled and loaded into the program: (1) written testimony against MAiD and (2) written testimony in support of MAiD. As the left side of figure 3.1 displays, individuals who testified against MAiD mobilized "suicide" and other affectively charged words, such as "lethal" and "kill," with comparatively high frequency. On the right side, we see that those in support of MAiD mobilized more benign terms such as "aid-in-dying," "option," and "end-of-life." These results suggest that the rebranding campaign described at the outset of this chapter may have resulted in further entrenchment of interlocutors' stances on MAiD. In other words, if you oppose MAiD, you are more likely to mobilize affectively charged legacy discourse, such as "assisted suicide," "kill," or "lethal." Meanwhile, MAiD proponents tend to rely on what Asen (2010) might call "strategic ambiguity," which is a way for interlocutors to "negotiate potentially competing situational demands, like multiple audiences with opposing interest" (p. 137). While proponents' strategic ambiguity was likely a well-meaning attempt at neutralizing the pathos-laden nature of the MAiD debate, it can also obscure stratified livability. To examine more closely whether and how death-with-dignity interlocutors were attuned to stratified livability, I had to do more than read from a distance. I needed to conduct a fine-grained analysis of MAiD testimony.

Second Analytic Approach: Summative Content Analysis

I relied on qualitative data analysis software (NVivo, version 12) to organize, categorize, and code data collected from both states' MAiD hearings, which included 537 forms of written testimony. First, I engaged in a rhetorically informed approach to "attribute coding" (Saldaña, 2013, p. 70), which enabled me to code each document for the following attributes:

- File type (e.g., meeting minutes, written testimony, amendments)
- State (i.e., Nevada, Connecticut)
- Hearing year (2017, 2019, 2021, 2022)
- Stance on MAiD (against, for, neutral)
- Positionality (e.g., state resident, health care provider, clergy, politician, lawyer)

When I examined how MAiD interlocutors' stances intersected with their self-stated positionality, I did not detect any obvious patterns (see appendix A). In other words, how one identified, professionally or otherwise, did not seem to correlate with a particular stance on MAiD, not even among clergy.

Given what I observed in the oral and written testimony of the hearings, and being initially unaware that utterances such as "death with dignity" were part of a tactical rebranding campaign (and not necessarily an official declaration), I then examined how dignity warranted state residents' stance on MAiD. To do that, I engaged in what might best be described as a kind of summative content analysis (Hseih & Shannon, 2005). I conducted a simple word search query to locate all instances of "dignity" across the whole corpus. By comparing the results of this query, I detected variation in how MAiD interlocutors mobilized dignity, which I documented by tagging testimony using three codes: dignity's rhetorical framing, dignity's adjacencies, and dignity's opposites.

Coding MAiD testimony for how interlocutors framed dignity (e.g., as a choice, idea, possession), situated dignity alongside adjacent values or concerns (e.g., autonomy, care, comfort), and situated dignity in opposition to certain concerns (e.g., embarrassment, fear, pain) allowed me to become familiar with deliberators' "end-of-life talk" (Segal, 2000a, p. 74). But not all death-with-dignity discourse was about the end of life. In fact, a good deal of testimony, especially among those who opposed MAiD, referenced their desire simply to live—that is, wanting to survive in an ableist world that seemingly did not want them there. The other pattern this analysis revealed was how shockingly insignificant "dignity" was in the MAiD testimony. Specifically, the word "dignity" appeared in only 177 of 537 forms of written testimony. And even then, dignity often occurred in the phrase "death with dignity" as a shorthand or vernacular substitute for the longer title of the state's MAiD bill. Dignity was not, counter to what I expected (or even hoped) to find, a meaningful intellectual warrant for residents' stance on MAiD. I started to suspect, therefore, that MAiD interlocutors who mobilized dignity did so as "mere rhetorical dressing" (Caulfield & Chapman, 2005, p. 737)—an otherwise unassuming verbal referent invoked as a commonplace and further evidence of "the universalist pretentions of Western humanism" (Mbembe, 2019, p. 161).

Because explicit references to dignity did little to reveal MAiD testimony's particularities, I needed to employ something more fine-grained than summative content analysis. A model for such fine-grained analysis exists in Pringle's (2019) "WPR method." The "WPR" portion of the method indexes the approach's central question: "What's the Problem Represented to Be?" Embedded in such an approach is the assumption that how a problem is framed as a problem—or what Pringle calls the "genealogical threads" that connect problematizations—favors "certain solutions" while precluding others (cf. Fairclough, 2013, p. 183). The WPR method traces how, according to Pringle, MAiD has evolved "from crime to care" (p. 3). What is more, discourses through which such genealogical threads can be traced "are not neutral, but instead are connected to cartographies of inequality" (Dutta, 2016, p. 17). To study genealogical threads, therefore, one must take a "culture-centered approach," which, in this chapter, means that I attend to the ways that death-with-dignity discourse emerges "at the intersections of structure and culture" (Dutta, p. 17).

Third Analytic Approach: Topological Analysis

Inspired by critical health communication's "culture-centered approach," I took a slightly different analytic tack by mobilizing the analytic power of a rhetorical lens—specifically, one that maps interlocutors' topological reasoning regarding their stance on MAiD. By "topological reasoning," I am referring to how interlocutors support their arguments with specific topoi. In addition to Hyde's definition provided earlier, I draw on Walsh and Boyle (2017), who argue that topologies articulate "the actors and arguments hiding in the unarticulated gaps and margins" (p. 10). Importantly, "*topoi* are Janus-faced," which, for my purposes, means that they are stance-agnostic (p. 10). In that same volume edited by Walsh and Boyle, I describe topological analyses as one way "to mine arguments" for their political and "value-laden conditions" (Teston, 2017b, p. 221). That is, topoi index common rhetorical premises on which both MAiD opponents and proponents hinge their arguments. For the purposes of this project, a word, phrase, or idea was characterized as a topos when it appeared in at least 50 MAiD opponents' or proponents' written testimonies.

Ultimately, my topological analysis of MAiD testimony identified seven core biopolitical topoi that MAiD interlocutors mobilized during hearings. In what follows, I illustrate the rhetorical function of each biopolitical topos by providing excerpts from written and spoken testimony. Although I am less interested in making claims about contemporary death-with-dignity discourse by quantifying articulations of stance on MAiD, appendix A indicates how stance and positionality broke down numerically in both states and during all four legislative years. In total, 272 forms of written testimony were opposed to MAiD; the remaining 259 forms of written testimony supported MAiD. Inspired by rhetoricians' premise that vernacular discourse reveals the contours of a controversy with greater specificity than do public opinion polls, I mention this breakdown to draw readers' attention to how different these numbers are from what public opinion polls find.[8] Once the Compassion & Choices form letters were removed from the corpus,[9] stance on MAiD was much more evenly distributed across those who opposed and those who supported the legislation. Polls obscure this even distribution.

Table 3.3 names the seven biopolitical topoi, defines them, and gives representative examples of how the topoi were mobilized by interlocutors on either side of the MAiD debate.[10] The seven biopolitical topoi are as follows: codes of conduct, cost, kinship, pain+control, precedent, safeguards, and vulnerability.

Table 3.4 displays how frequently the seven biopolitical topoi were mobilized by either MAiD opponents or proponents. Notice the two biopolitical topoi in the shaded rows: *cost* and *vulnerability*. The cost and vulnerability topoi are distinctive from the other five in that they were referenced significantly more frequently by those who opposed MAiD than by those who supported it. Specifically, cost appeared in 113 of 272 MAiD opponents' written testimony, while it appeared in only 38 of 259 MAiD proponents' written testimony. Vulnerability, too, had nearly a 2:1 ratio in the corpora, with 100 MAiD opponents mobilizing the topos versus only 46 MAiD proponents. For the other five biopolitical topoi, both sides of the MAiD debate mobilized them with similar frequency (oppose vs. support): codes of conduct (85 vs. 71), kinship (116 vs. 144), pain+control (122 vs. 150), precedent (82 vs. 78), and safeguards (60 vs. 58). In other words, opponents used these five topoi about as often as proponents did. These five are what I see as "topological commonplaces" in that interlocutors on both sides of the debate seemed to prefer the rhetorical affordances they offered. In what follows, I detail first how the topological commonplaces functioned in MAiD testimony; I then explain how cost and vulnerability functioned as topological divergences.

TABLE 3.3.

Biopolitical topoi, *definitions, and examples from MAiD testimony*

Biopolitical topos	Definition	Examples (paraphrased)	
		Oppositional stance	Supportive stance
Codes of conduct	Reference to an explicit, often institutionally sanctioned, expectation for how to act	Religious/spiritual beliefs; Hippocratic Oath's "do no harm" mandate; integrity of the medical profession	Constitution's separation of church and state; Nuremburg Code, Declaration of Helsinki's four pillars of medical ethics; medical "standards of care"
Cost	Concern about limited material or financial resources	Health care's cost will encourage insurance companies to ration care	Health care's cost will result in increased debt
Kinship	Reference to the (absent or present) role of family, friends, and other loved ones	No kin makes someone vulnerable; family needs to spend time with a dying member; family could have ulterior motives	Family is forced to witness suffering otherwise; protracted illness burdens family members; increased conversation with family about end-of-life wishes
Pain+Control	Attempt to resolve tension between how an individual experiences their pain and who/what decides when a certain level of pain is permissible	Right to bodily autonomy, choice, and self-determination; gives doctors too much power; gives the state too much power; existing measures (e.g., hospice and advanced directives) already work; right to die becomes duty to die	Pain and (anticipatory) suffering are mitigated by the "placebo effect" that comes from having the option of ending one's life; a human being's natural right to die; bodily autonomy (e.g., bowels, breathing)
Precedent	Reference to a model of one or more extant (often quantifiable) practices	Suicide contagion; the Netherlands	Oregon; public support for legislation; existing right to other freedoms (gun ownership, etc.); euthanasia of pets as analog
Safeguards	Reference to some aspect of the proposed legislation that legally safeguards against an aforementioned concern about MAiD	The safeguards will not be good enough	The safeguards will be good enough
Vulnerability	Explicit invocation of first- or secondhand knowledge about a vulnerable person's experience	Concern about disabled persons and the elderly	Generic references to "our most vulnerable"

TABLE 3.4.
Frequency of biopolitical topoi relative to MAiD stance in written testimony

Biopolitical topos	Oppositional stance (n = 272)	Supportive stance (n = 259)
Codes of conduct	85	71
Cost	113	38
Kinship	116	144
Pain+Control	122	150
Precedent	82	78
Safeguards	60	58
Vulnerability	100	46
TOTAL	**229**	**207**

Topological Commonplace #1: Codes of Conduct

Written testimony was coded as *codes of conduct* when someone explicitly referenced an institutionally sanctioned expectation for how to act. Such an expectation might include a religious doctrine, professional standard, or a political/legal declaration, for example. As Battin (2005) rightly identified in her "paradigmatic argument-scheme about physician-assisted suicide," MAiD opponents did, indeed, offer testimony premised on religious doctrine. It was common to hear testimony that positioned God as the ultimate choice-maker: "God holds us in the palm of his hand. Life and death are His to give and to take in His time, wisdom, love, and mercy." But even those who wrote in support of MAiD occasionally deferred to religious doctrine. In other words, religion as a code of conduct was not unique to MAiD opponents' logic. In such cases, what MAiD proponents highlighted was a divinely bestowed power of free will: "Life is a God-given right—but so is also free will. That was a the [*sic*] greatest gift that God gave us—the ability to choose for ourselves."

The spectrum of institutionally sanctioned expectations for how to act also included, again as one might expect, professional standards. For example, one MAiD opponent referenced the American Medical Association's Code of Medical Ethics, which states that "permitting physicians to engage in assisted suicide would ultimately cause more harm than good." Like their opposition, MAiD proponents also invoked professional standards, this time from the Connecticut Nurses Association: "CNA believes that SB 88 is in alignment with our professional position statement and code of ethics to support the professional nurse in advocating for a patient's right to self-determination while providing sufficient safeguards for all involved in these complex matters." Here we see evidence of what Phillips (2009) found in a study of how "assisted suicide" was navigated by certain health professions. Phillips described a tension that nurses, in particular, must navigate: in cases where a patient is at the end of life, nurses embody care in the interstices—the space between what Phillips names "the personal desires of patients" and "the medical imperative of the physician" (p. 148). So, while the topos of codes of conduct was the least surprising of the seven, it hardly settles the debate for one side or the other. Logics of care/lessness premised on codes of conduct—whether religious, professional, or legal—were modulated by testimony that valued the opposite end of the individual–institutional spectrum, including references to moving stories about loved ones' experiences with death and dying. These logics were what I termed "kinship," which I discuss next.

Topological Commonplace #2: Kinship

Written testimony was coded *kinship* when someone explicitly referenced the role of family, friends, or other loved ones as part of their stance on MAiD. Both sides recounted dozens of firsthand experiences with a mother, father, aunt, uncle, sister, or brother for whom MAiD was either a threat or a godsend.[11]

In addition to telling moving stories about a relative or loved one's dying experience, some MAiD oppositionists mobilized kinship arguments to argue for the value of prolonging the dying experience. The line of reasoning was that prolonging the dying experience enabled, at least for some, more time for the family to heal and experience a sense of closure. One husband described how the slow death of his wife, Judith, which included "times of treatment, pain, and growing physical weakness," enabled him to witness "Judith's relationship with God intensify, our marriage grow and . . . relationship with our children and grandchildren blossom." Here and elsewhere, kinship's topological suasiveness emerged alongside assumptions about a so-called natural death and dying process, which presumably meant not using modern medicine (including the lethal cocktail of pharmaceuticals prescribed for MAiD patients) to intervene in the process: "true compassion and dignity" involved "wanting to walk along with them . . . through a natural dying process." For some opponents, MAiD was an actual *threat* to familial closeness: "Surrogates, family members and friends, and beneficiaries will all be plunged into controversy, confusion, ambivalence and guilt as this planned death rolls forward."

Interlocutors on both sides similarly cited a wide range of personal and heartfelt experiences they'd had while watching a family member die. Here is one example: "Her devastating diagnosis of ALS came in February 2009 and she deteriorated at an astonishing rate. She wanted the same kind of peaceful end that my father had experienced and had told me she hoped the end would come quickly." Similarly, a social worker who testified in support of MAiD reported that she often witnessed families and friends suffer because of a loved one's prolonged death:

> As a Clinical Social Worker with 35 years' experience, I have seen many clients and their families who have needed to care for a terminally ill family member or close friend. I have seen the emotional impact on them as they attend to loved ones who are suffering with a degenerative disease when those loved ones have clearly asked for aid with the process of dying. Their feelings of anguish, powerlessness and helplessness often contribute to higher-than-normal levels of depression and anxiety. This experience has led me to support a terminally ill patient's right to choose to end their suffering by getting the support and assistance they need to allow them die peacefully.

Often, when MAiD proponents referenced a desire for dying "peacefully" among family and friends, they also invoked the importance of "dying at home." For example, one health care provider (HCP) made the case that her "family, friends, and patients . . . want a peaceful ending, surrounded by loved ones, not strangers and fluorescent lighting, and beeping machines." A Las Vegas resident with multiple myeloma made a similar case but added a religiously inspired codes of conduct topos to that of kinship:

> Doctors gave me five years to live. I am not afraid of what comes next as I prepare to live what doctors say is the last year of my life. For now, I continue to undergo different types of treatments to have a better quality of

> life. But the blood cancer is taking a toll on my body. I am tired. I am in pain. I have a lesion in my neck. I am scared. My focus is to live my last days surrounded by my four adult children and two grandbabies. I do not want to be connected to machines, catheters and tubes that will cause more pain and vomiting that will only debilitate my body. When my Lord calls me, I want to die peacefully, surrounded by my husband and our two sons, two daughters and our precious grandchildren . . . holding my hand in prayer.

Although dying at home around loved ones was framed as desirable by folks on both sides of the MAiD debate, Braswell (2011) notes that hospice patients without family or primary caretakers "are left at home," sometimes "in conditions that are negligent or abusive" (p. 76). In fact, "the U.S. hospice system systematically discriminates against terminally ill patients without kinship support" (Braswell, p. 77). Dominant discourse in the MAiD debate, then, seems to obscure the particularities of certain persons' kinship status. An indifference to difference emerges. That is, concern for the importance of (presumably biological) family, while prioritized by both sides, "discriminates against" those "who do not have primary caretakers" (Braswell, p. 76), those whose home situation is abusive, or those whose kinship networks, due to finances or other reasons, are unable to enact the kind of kinship that is normatively idealized in MAiD testimony.

Topological Commonplace #3: Pain+Control

The third topological commonplace, *pain+control*, is a slightly modified version of Battin's proposition, namely, that at the heart of MAiD proponents' reasoning are two distinct concerns: pain and autonomous control. My analyses show that rather than two distinct concerns, pain and control are tethered in contemporary death-with-dignity discourse. Again, both MAiD proponents *and* opponents relied on topological premises involving who had the power or agency to manage corporeal pain in a particular way. The pain+control topos is where I locate testimony that saw the solution to corporeal pain as an idealized, universal notion of individual choice or self-determination.[12] In such discourse, interlocutors attempted to persuade their audience of the jurisdictional constraints associated with governing the body at the end of life, including managing pain and suffering.[13]

Questions that interlocutors attempted to answer when mobilizing the pain+control topos included these, for example: Are pain and suffering required parts of the human experience that everyone must endure? Should physicians have the power to decide when enough pain and suffering have occurred? Do individual patients have a right to decide, even before experiencing pain and suffering, to hasten their death? What is the role of the state in resolving the tension between an individual's experience of pain and their bodily autonomy? Interlocutors on both sides of the MAiD debate grappled with these questions equally, with a slight proclivity among those who supported the bill to mobilize the "patients' rights" argument. Notably, a handful of Nevadans mobilized the pain+control topos by questioning the role of the state in influencing these matters at all—that is, some critiqued the state's attempt at making laws that "establish the supremacy of the state in life and death decisions" (McDorman, 2005, p. 257). Some MAiD proponents used the pain+control topos to call out "government interference" in one's "right to die," while MAiD opponents brought up pain+control in describing how dangerous it was for the government to legislate death and dying at all, noting that the "right to die" could become a "duty to die."

Those who wrote to oppose MAiD attempted to resolve the tension between pain and control by reminding readers that it is within a person's right to refuse (excessive) medical intervention. In some cases, this was referred to as "comfort care": "Many people think assisted suicide is necessary to prevent agonizing pain, but attentive comfort care—now this is a right to insist on!—can control pain in dying patients, through palliative sedation if necessary. And people have had the long-standing right to refuse any treatment, including food and water." A more extreme version of this argument was that persons can always elect, in an advance directive (a legal document stipulating a person's wishes about life-extending medical intervention should they later become mentally incompetent), not to be resuscitated or intubated. Notably, however, health communication researchers have pointed out how even a patient's advance directive can sometimes be overridden in certain circumstances, thereby shifting who has control at the end of life. MAiD testimony was sensitive to this reality and argued that such legislation would further empower health care professionals to control how and when a patient died: "[MAiD] does not give more power to patients, it gives it to doctors. Do we really want to give this power to our physicians?"

In response to MAiD opponents' concern over power and control at the end of life, some proponents expressed outrage: "Oh my God, what the Hell are these God Damn perverts thinking? That everyone should suffer like this, and not have a choice to die with less pain and more dignity?" For many MAiD proponents, a patient's control over their body—autonomy—was what mattered most: "Medical aid in dying legislation like House Bill 6425 will provide terminally-ill individuals like my Aunt [redacted] the opportunity to quickly end their pain and suffering at the very end of life, through the use of safe and reliable medical means, entirely on their own terms, and avoid prolonged suffering. Our country is founded on the fundamental notion that we as individuals are free to choose how to live their lives, and that necessarily includes the right to choose how we die."

While not everyone situated choice and self-determination in (liberal humanist) American values, or "nationalistic discourses" (Hamraie, 2017, p. 72), self-determination was central to MAiD proponents' logic of care/lessness. And for some pro-MAiD residents, self-determination didn't always result in someone actually ingesting the life-ending medication. Here, MAiD was discursively framed as having what some interlocuters called a "placebo effect." That is, even if an individual did not take the prescribed life-ending medication, "simply having the option available, in and of itself, offers solace." Signaling the importance of autonomous control at the end of life, pro-MAiD testimony highlighted how in states where MAiD is legal, "many of them [patients] don't even use the medication, instead getting comfort in the idea that they alone have control over their destiny."

Topological Commonplace #4: Precedent

Written testimony was coded *precedent* when an individual identified one or more extant patterns or practices as a model to emulate. The spectrum of precedent-based arguments ranged from laws and practices in specific geographic regions (including countries outside the United States) to precedent-setting propositions derived from scientific studies. Those who wrote to oppose MAiD frequently invoked warnings about the Netherlands, for example: "Consider that the Netherlands—a country which has a longstanding practice of euthanasia and assisted suicide—recently found not guilty of murder a doctor who euthanized a patient with dementia against her will." Opponents also invoked precedent to call into question the hypocrisy of such legislation, as states with a MAiD law had failed to reduce suicide rates: "The United States has been struggling the past many years with ever increasing teen suicides. Although all States have suffered with the tragedy of teen suicide, Oregon's increase has been disproportionate." Here, opponents mobilized as part of the precedent-based argument the assumption that suicide rates and the legalization of MAiD are correlated (from a logic of "suicide contagion").

Meanwhile, those who supported MAiD frequently invoked other states' supposed success with such legislation: "With more than 60 years of combined experience across ten authorized jurisdictions, we have conclusive evidence that medical aid in dying has not resulted in any unintended negative consequences." The assumption here is that what counts as success in one state will count as success in all states. There is little if any accounting, in other words, for the ways that specific living conditions and forms of state support may affect death and dying at the end of life. In addition to other states' practices and public opinion polls, some MAiD proponents went as far as to mobilize as precedent *veterinary* standards of care. Repeatedly I read testimony that cited the widely accepted practice of pet euthanasia in the United States as grounds for passing MAiD legislation: "The fact that we allow this kind of inhumane suffering, the kind that we don't even allow our pets to endure, is shameful." Here, the pain+control topos intersects with precedent (albeit among veterinary medicine) to further flatten varying vulnerability—this time even between human animals and nonhuman animals.

Topological Commonplace #5: Safeguards

The final topological commonplace was *safeguards*, this study's only "in vivo code," in the terms of Saldaña (2013, p. 4). Written testimony was coded for the presence of a safeguard assertion when an individual cited an aspect of the proposed legislation that would enable or fail to enable a legal "safeguard" that should protect against some concern about MAiD. In two examples taken from opponents' testimony, interlocuters claimed the legislation would leave some safeguards open to circumvention (emphasis added):

> Other ostensible *safeguards* are overcome by doctor-shopping, which this bill makes easier than previous versions by allowing the attending and consulting physicians to work together in the same office.

> Due to the overly broad definitions of attending and consulting physician, there is no *safeguard* to prevent out of state, rubber stamp physicians to be used in Nevada, which in turn, makes it virtually impossible to effectively monitor a physician's behavior to prevent abuses. Since there is no independent qualified monitor, there is no way of knowing that the patient knowingly and voluntarily administered the lethal dose, let alone whether there were complications from the death drug. The potential of abuse by unscrupulous heirs will go unchecked. The lack of a residency definition will allow suicide tourism.

Meanwhile, those who supported MAiD warranted their stance by mobilizing the significance of the bills' safeguards, which required (among other things) that individuals orally self-administer the lethal medication: "No other person, including the qualified patient themselves, may administer the medication by intravenous injection or infusion. This is an important safeguard in assuring patients always maintain decision making authority and are able to change their minds at any time." Notably, the oral "self-administration" safeguard would disadvantage patients who cannot orally self-administer medication, as is the case for some patients with amyotrophic lateral sclerosis.

As a kind of ethos-building move, the safeguards topos also enabled MAiD proponents to demonstrate that they were responsive to opponents' concerns. As similar bills had previously made their way through other states' legislatures, lawmakers in Nevada and Connecticut learned from those states' MAiD deliberations. Authors of the proposed bills in Nevada and Connecticut, therefore, had drafted explicit safeguards in anticipation of obstacles that other states had encountered during deliberations. Other states' concerns that the proposed bills attempted to safeguard against were matters such as who would be listed as the cause of death on the death certificate, who must or can be present during self-administration of the lethal medication, and how does one demonstrate they are of sound mind when requesting MAiD. Proponents' appeals to safeguards aimed not only to set others' minds at ease about the presumed protective power of the law, but they also signified to their opposition, "we hear you." For example:

> Those opponents advance heartfelt concerns, such as the risk for coercion and elder abuse; worrying whether individuals will be subject to a premature death should the 6 month estimate of life expectancy prove to be inaccurate; the insistence that insurance companies will force patients to utilize medical aid in dying because they won't pay for continued medical care; or the slippery slope that expands eligibility for medical aid in dying beyond the scope of criteria explicitly listed in this House Bill. While these concerns are undoubtedly sincere, they ignore considerable *safeguards* built into H. B. 6425. (emphasis added)

One way to read the above testimony is as a kind of considerate gesture that honors the sincere concerns of one's opponents. Another way to read it is as a patronizing if not naïve disregard for how even the most explicit legislative safeguard cannot fully protect patients who are varyingly vulnerable. In her critique of the ways epigenetic science, for example, further reifies the harms caused previously by genetic racism, Jackson (2020) argues that "systemic racism . . . exceeds the health safeguards class mobility would presumably provide and regulation purports to protect" (p. 206). MAiD testimony from "precarious publics" (Teston et al., 2019) similarly emphasized how legal safeguards could not, as Jackson describes, protect them from necropolitical logics.

This brings me to the two final biopolitical topoi, cost and vulnerability. Even though these two topoi are employed in testimony from both sides of the MAiD debate, I have labeled them "topological divergences" because one side (opponents) overwhelmingly preferred these topoi, while the other side did not. Among these two topological divergences are some of the same un/dignified asides described in chapter two.

Topological Divergence #1: Cost

When an individual explained their stance on MAiD by expressing concern about limited material or financial resources, such a concern was coded *cost*. This topos was one of two that were mobilized significantly more frequently by MAiD opponents. References to cost appeared in 113 opponents' written testimony but in only 38 proponents' written testimony. The topos of cost was often accompanied by appeals not to "be a burden"—a sentiment expressed, as you may recall, in chapter two by some of Naomi's patients. For example, "When people do not have access to paid in-home caregivers, they are susceptible to feeling like a burden." Implicit in this individual's testimony against MAiD was a structural critique of the US health care system like that which I described in the previous chapter. Persons who could not afford to pay for home visits from HCPs, who would aid with bathing and other core care functions, often ended up having to call on family and friends for help. Even if, in a perfect world, one's family and friends are happy to help their loved one, "compulsory able-bodiedness" (McRuer, 2010, p. 369) and even "able-mindedness" (Kafer, 2013, p. 184) are so endemic to US culture that dying persons still described feeling like a financial burden.[14] And as we saw in the previous chapter, cost-based logics of care/lessness are distributed across the entirety of the caretaking apparatus, including and especially in insurance companies.

One interlocutor married cost with the kinship topos in asking, "Will the desire to spare relatives or to preserve family resources create a sense of obligation—perhaps even a duty—to die sooner rather than later?" Similarly, another MAiD opponent observed, "the starved patient could be influenced to view 'aid in dying' as the best way out of an intolerable situation, or believe her family would be better off without her emotionally and financially." Opponents were especially keen to mobilize the cost topos by citing shocking claims about insurance companies that allegedly denied expensive medical treatments and, in their place, recommended MAiD. Much like Karen Ann Quinlan's and Terri Schiavo's names continue to circulate as "rhetorical icons" within death-with-dignity discourse (Kenny, 2005, p. 17), so too did certain patients' names that had been published in local newspapers in stories about insurance companies' profit-driven practices (see also Hyde & McSpiritt, 2007). Here is one instance: "Last summer, seriously-ill Californian Stephanie Packer received a letter from her insurer refusing to cover a prescribed course of chemotherapy. Meanwhile, she was told that her co-pay for just-legalized assisted suicide would be $1.20. Congress is now in the process of trying to repeal the Affordable Care Act, threatening millions with loss of insurance. Because assisted suicide will always be the cheapest treatment, short- and long-term, its availability will inevitably affect medical decision-making." Some version of the Stephanie Packer story appeared in three forms of written testimony and was mentioned by participants in the 2017 Nevada hearing and the 2021 Connecticut hearing. Such stories not only hinge on the precedent topos described above, but they also paint a damning picture of a heartless health care system that would rather let people die than spend money to keep them alive.

Other MAiD opponents expanded their indictment of insurance companies' profit-driven practices to include doctors and hospitals: "People are denied coverage because insurance companies look for profit, not for the welfare of the patient (their customer). Medical institutions, individual doctor practices and hospitals are businesses, also concerned with profit. Research is stymied because funding is not available." Attuned to the reality of un/dignified asides, one interlocuter was unafraid to make cost connections between contemporary COVID-19 constraints and MAiD: "At the beginning of this pandemic, discussions were had in ethical circles of how to treat people with scarce resources and who gets those scarce resources. If this bill passes, do requests for aid-in-dying and subsequent possession of lethal medication become factors in determining whether or not the 'qualified patient' receives medical resources—scarce or not? Could such a 'qualified patient' be denied medical resources? Yes. It [resource rationing] has already happened before."

Concern about resource rationing was prevalent among MAiD oppositionists long before COVID-19, though. In fact, some HCPs who were well versed in the Physicians for Compassionate Care Education Foundation's interpretation of the health plan of Oregon (where MAiD is legal) cited a list of "prioritized services" for patients who are near the end of life. According to the foundation, such services include MAiD but not chemotherapy, surgical interventions, or "medical equipment or supplies which will not benefit the patient for a reasonable length of time." The cost topos was also mobilized as a rebuttal to some MAiD proponents' pain+control arguments by inviting the audience to consider how profitability was a factor in many end-of-life efforts at controlling pain.

Other opponents employed the cost topos to call into question the fact that enacting MAiD was being deliberated at all. One individual complained, "Why are legislators wasting time, money, and resources with this bill? We have other more immediate and pressing problems in CT, including an opioid crisis, a severe lack of services for mental health patients, increasing crime, and billions of dollars of unfunded liabilities." Another individual who described MAiD as "state sponsored suicide" accused MAiD sponsors of repeatedly attempting "to coerce the public and abuse taxpayer resources."

Whether it was an accusation of misusing taxpayers' or insurance companies' resources, concerns about cost appeared disproportionally important among those who opposed MAiD. But cost-based logics of care/lessness appeared in pro-MAiD testimony too, albeit sparingly. What is interesting is that pro-MAiD testimony that mobilized the cost topos invoked some of the same concerns that opponents raised—specifically, concerns about becoming a financial burden: "I certainly don't want to burden my family with unnecessary and horrendous medical bills should I become either physically or mentally incapacitated, let alone burden them with the mental and physical trauma of having to deal with the issue. I would like to know that I had the legal choice to choose death over the indignities of an extended life that medical technology has now made available." Adjacent to concerns about cost were references to individuals' fears of becoming "physically or mentally incapacitated," as the passage above demonstrates." One's incapacitation—for reasons related to age or disability—animates the final topos, vulnerability.

Topological Divergence #2: Vulnerability

The concept of vulnerability is fraught with ambiguity. But for my purposes, I'm drawing on Oliviero's (2018) contention that "vulnerability is more a *subjectivity* and *political context* rather than an identity" (p. 47; emphasis in the original). More to the point, Oliviero argues that while vulnerability "may be a universal ontological condition . . . it is also experienced unequally and shifts in a way that both clings to and exceeds identity-based categories" (p. 47). MAiD testimony was coded *vulnerability* when an individual warranted their stance on MAiD by explicitly invoking a vulnerable encounter experienced either by themselves or by another person. References to vulnerability appeared in 100 MAiD opponents' written testimony and only 46 MAiD proponents' written testimony. It is in this topological divergence that we see MAiD's potential consequences for people whose bodies do not fit within the "normate template" I referenced in chapter one (Hamraie, 2017, p. 19).

For example, one MAiD opponent asked committee members "to put yourselves in the shoes of ordinary people of color, disabled people and the elderly who struggle to be seen as full persons in the health care system." Another opponent appealed to the vulnerability status to "our elderly," who "will be pressured with a duty to die or open obvious pathways for abuse." In addition to elder abuse, there was even a sensitivity to economic class among MAiD opponents who mobilized vulnerability arguments: "Assisted suicide endangers all terminal patients. It puts a disproportionate pressure on people with disabilities and the economically disadvantaged, leaving a great many with suicide being the only 'treatment' to which they have equal access." This topos vividly demonstrates how "policies often enact and enforce symbolic hierarchies that unite and divide people . . . policies can bring people together . . . and policies can pull people apart, constituting some individuals and groups as 'other' and inferior to conventional practices and beliefs" (Asen, 2010, pp. 127–128). The vulnerability topos drew attention to how MAiD legislation assumed an able-bodied, "unmarked," and "privileged" dying patient (Happe, 2013, p. 148).

Here again, MAiD opponents were inspired to draw on COVID-19 conditions as backing for their vulnerability arguments. That's what "the last year" meant in one interlocuter's testimony: "The last year has given us terrible insight into the ageist and ableist country we are—one which treats the old and disabled like throwaway populations, discarded into warehouses of death. We've also seen how terribly we treat those with dementia in particular, and the thousands and thousands of 'excess deaths' of this population during the pandemic is too awful to contemplate." Here and elsewhere, the vulnerability topos highlights how MAiD legislation seeds the "authorized disposability" of "the old and disabled" (Jackson, 2016, p. 19).

To be fair, at least one MAiD proponent did offer support for the bill contingent on their concern for "vulnerable populations": "It is critical that the legislature consult with disability rights groups to make sure the bill allows people their individual right to determine when to end their life but also closes any loopholes that could hurt vulnerable populations." Although it is unlikely to be intentionally malicious, this line of reasoning compares concerns about treating disabled persons "like throwaway populations" to mere loopholes. To such seemingly benign, yet normalized indignity, we might reply with Mol's (2021) admonition: "Situations in which complexity stands out call instead for a genre of *doing* where good intentions are always combined with attentive inquiries into potential adverse effects" (p. 99).

Pro-MAiD testimony that mobilized the vulnerability topos employed a more common pattern, though: ventriloquizing and rebutting the opposition:[15]

> I also understand the reasons why the disabled community is worried about MAID's possible effect on its members. However, there is little evidence in this country, in the states where MAID is legal, that any slippery slope has occurred.

> It's important to note that advanced age, disability and chronic health conditions are not qualifying factors for medical aid in dying.

> These scare tactics include concerns the law would target the disabled, elderly, frail, uninsured and other vulnerable groups.

MAiD proponents also employed the vulnerability topos when they critiqued disabled persons for being hysterical and spreading misinformation: "Very much like the anti-vaccine community, the vocal disability rights community is well funded, very vocal, but also very small. They are not representative of the broader disabled community. Surveys show that 65% of disabled voters in Connecticut favor Aid in Dying legislation. Much like the anti-vaccine argument, the argument from this vocal minority is one of fear and misinformation. The fear is understandable. The misinformation is unforgivable."

Contrary to what some pro-MAiD testimony suggested, concerns about cost and vulnerability from people that the above individual called a "vocal minority" aren't manufactured hysteria. More than 25% of people with disabilities in the United States live below the poverty line. Even if disabled persons were, in fact, a vocal minority, the implicit assumption that it would be impractical to try and shape policy in response to their concerns is carelessness in action.

When MAiD proponents were not ventriloquizing or gaslighting their opposition, they occasionally leveraged the vulnerability topos to point out their own personal experiences with being disabled and/or terminally ill. For example,

> The past year I underwent a triple bypass and experienced two strokes that have been debilitating. In the past 12 years I have survived late stage cancer and undergone many preventative surgeries to avoid hereditary cancer to vulnerable organs in order to preserve and to extend life, my colon, female organs, gall bladder and breasts. I cherish life, however during that time, I laid in bed for months in institutional health settings, and found it offered extensive time to consider the future. I do not wish to live that way, in older age, writhing in pain and unable to complete even my own basic needs.

Here, the experience of being institutionalized warranted one interlocuter's supportive stance on MAiD while disarming the opposition. Testimony such as this, though, not only works through empathic logics of "abstract intimacy" (Berlant), but it also pathologizes dependency (Oliviero, 2018, p. 253).

Rather than pathologizing dependency—with reference, in the quotation above, to an inability "to complete even my own basic needs"—an opportunity for interdependence emerges. A compelling description of interdependence can be found in Eli Clare's (2017) *Brilliant Imperfection*:

> White Western culture goes to extraordinary lengths to deny the vital relationships between water and stone, plant and animal, human and nonhuman, as well as the utter reliance of human upon human. Within this

> culture of denial, when those of us who don't currently need help dressing ourselves or going to the bathroom try to imagine interdependence, we fail. In conjuring a world where we need care to get up in the morning and go to bed at night, we picture an overwhelming dependency, a terrifying loss of privacy and dignity. We don't pause to notice that our fears reflect not the truth but the limits of our imagination. (p. 136)

Here, Clare uncovers another premise upon which the pathologizing of inter/dependency hinges: a lack of imagination.

In each vulnerability assertion quoted from MAiD proponents, we see one of at least two kinds of ableist responses: "one might pity them. One may, on the other hand, respond to them with hostility" (Reynolds, 2022, p. 124). But interlocuters against MAiD who mobilized vulnerability were careful to confront pitiful or hostile responses: "We disabled people have lives that frequently look like the lives of people requesting assisted suicide, but we reject the prejudice that personal dignity is somehow lost through physical dependence on others, or because we are not continent every hour of every day." Another MAiD opponent who identified as disabled rebutted MAiD proponents' argument that "life in a wheelchair" conferred a "loss of autonomy" and "being a burden on others." Instead, she called out MAiD proponents' vulnerability arguments for promoting "systemic ableism that gives the message that depending on the care of others, as often happens in the aging process or by having a disability, is a fate worse than others." This testimony illustrates how dominant discourse around MAiD legislation pathologizes dependency. Pathologized dependency is eugenic logics' inner kernel.

Critiques of pathologized dependency were threaded through many MAiD opponents' vulnerability arguments that addressed past and present racist, ableist, and ageist practices:

> It [MAiD] increases the tendency for medical personnel to make judgements about their patient's quality of life and if they deserve treatment. The truth is, we do it now! Implicit bias has been studied at length and we know that it affects patient care. Studies show that minorities often receive different treatment and disabled people will testify to prejudice in their care. With DPS, attitudes will change. If patient A has done the "noble thing" by taking his life, why is patient B still here when his care is so

> physically and financially taxing? The so called right to die will become a duty to die.

Because medical racism (or what the testimony above calls "implicit bias") is an "undignified aside," it was rarely mentioned during MAiD testimony. But some form of concern about "patient B" in the testimony cited above appeared in almost half of MAiD opponents' written testimony. By confronting how the vulnerability topos was inappropriately yoked with the pain+control topos to produce pathologized dependency, those opposed to the bill alerted their audience to MAiD legislation's (implicit) message: "When assisted suicide proponents assert that losing one's autonomy or becoming a burden on family or having no dignity because of the inability to feed oneself constitutes reasons for committing assisted suicide, people with disabilities remind everyone that such reasons describe the disabled; and if society accepts such reasons as valid for causing death by assisted suicide, the message is sent—intended or not, like it or not—that the disabled would be better off dead as well." To be clear, not all persons with disabilities testified in opposition to MAiD. But consistently, in each hearing I analyzed, there existed a concern, whether explicit or in the background, that the logics of care/lessness upon which MAiD legislation rested were rooted in pathologized dependency.

I conclude my analysis by highlighting how some of the most persuasive testimony against MAiD came from those who represented or identified as disabled US veterans.[16] One example at a Connecticut hearing came from Mr. Sherman Gillums Jr.[17] At one point he broke from his script to rebut the ableism in a previous person's testimony in which a man had bemoaned the fact that, without MAiD, his wife would have "been in a wheelchair for the rest of her life." Mr. Gillums, a Black US veteran and wheelchair user responded, "You know what? *I am in a wheelchair for the rest of my life*. And it's a pretty dignified life that I live right now." As an especially effective rhetor, Mr. Gillums mobilized all seven biopolitical topoi in his written testimony:

- codes of conduct (via the Hippocratic Oath): "This bill would turn the definition of 'humane' on its head by depersonalizing accountability among physicians to 'do no harm' while legitimizing one form of suicide, under the guise of medical practice, and failing to distinguish it from the act of using a firearm or other lethal means to end depression or hopelessness."

- cost: "Assisted suicide would create perverse incentives for insurance companies to deny care to patients and offer death instead. This fear is not based on theory or a slippery slope fallacy."
- kinship: "My grandmother died from a terminal blood cancer in 2010. I don't take her suffering or the suffering of others lightly. She was in extreme pain until her dying day, and it hurt my family to see that."
- pain+control: "The argument here is not that people should be talked into living in pain based on some philosophical notion that self-killing is wrong . . . It is not a physician's job to deliberately end a human life, even when that life appears hopeless to the one who is living it, which is precisely why we have palliative care to address humanely end-of-life health matters."
- precedent: "After Brittany Maynard, who was diagnosed with an astrocytoma and became a highly visible spokesperson for the legalization of physician-assisted death, died by lethal ingestion in Oregon in 2014, the publicly-available data revealed that in the months surrounding Maynard's high-profile death, the number of similarly situated individuals in Oregon who ended their lives by lethal ingestion more than doubled."
- safeguards: "The bill also takes great care to include provisions on informed consent, freedom from coercion or undue influence, and criminal penalties in instances where an assisted death results from wrongful activity, which at least give it the appearance of a humane piece of legislation—with emphasis on appearance."
- vulnerability: "In closing, what H.B. 6425 will do is essentially demean those who die by suicide for other reasons, which include the consequences of fighting our Nation's wars . . ."

I chose to feature Mr. Gillums's words not just because they powerfully and persuasively illustrate each of this study's seven biopolitical topoi. Mr. Gillums's words also "make us think and care about what we say and do," as his words call "for acknowledgment" (Hyde, 2006, p. 141). I see Mr. Gillums offering more than just a discursive takedown of his opposition's reasoning. He embodies "how people who are being marginalized and experiencing a social death" might be acknowledged legislatively (Hyde, 2006, p. 85–86). Mr. Gillums's testimony illustrates how public policy risks normalizing stratified livability. His testimony foregrounds "how some groups are more systematically exposed to precariousness than others" (Oliviero, 2018, p. 47).

Physical disability, as Mr. Gillums's testimony illustrates, intersects with a range of other identities and material-discursive factors, including mental health, class, genetics, professional power differentials, and geopolitical conflict. The intersection of class, race, and disability is a precarious one that deserves acknowledgment when deliberating not just about death and dying but also about how to discern between dying and living in the first place. Much of pro-MAiD testimony reflected what Iris Marion Young (1997) describes as "unconscious assumptions and reactions of well-meaning people in ordinary interactions" (p. 41). When combined with "media and cultural stereotypes" as well as "bureaucratic hierarchies and market mechanisms," or what she calls "the normal processes of everyday life" (p. 21), it's easy to see how unconscious ableist assumptions and reactions scale up to necropolitical policies and practices.

Results from my analysis suggest that state legislators charged with making decisions about life and death need to develop "cultural competence" (Garland-Thomson, 2017b, p. 325), learn how to de-medicalize disability (p. 327), and resist necropolitical logics of care/lessness that hinge on compulsory able-bodiedness (McRuer, 2010). Price (2015) takes such resistance a step further by advocating instead for disability as *desirable*: "scarred skin is beauty; slurred speech is music; the tapping of a cane is power" (p. 275). Indeed, "being witnessed and cared for" was often missing in MAiD hearings as residents were limited to five minutes of speaking time (Price, p. 280).

As Mr. Gillums and other MAiD critics demonstrate, the MAiD debate can no longer be characterized as a debate only about pain relief or religious conviction. And I'm not even sure we can still assert, as Hyde does, that controversies such as MAiD are decided by those who end up telling the best stories. Good stories were told by folks on both sides of the MAiD debate. We need to examine critically the biopolitical topoi that make a story sound good to begin with. The paradigm shift required for responding ethically to MAiD critics' arguments grounded in cost and vulnerability requires legislators (and state residents) to at least "think disability otherwise" (Kafer, 2014, p. 153), if not come to desire it (Price, 2015, p. 275)—that is, to resee disability as something other than "an individual tragedy or misfortune due to genetic or environmental insult" (Reynolds, 2022, p. 7). These are ableist logics that fortify "eugenic discourses and practices" (Reynolds, p. 6). These same logics also fortify "legal constructions of subjects who are in need of state 'protection,'" which is yet another form of pathologized dependency (Oliviero, 2018, p. 50). Over time, pathologized dependency scales up to stratified livability.

MAiD legislation, therefore, exists "at the deadly intersection of medical abandonment and overexposure" (Benjamin, 2016, p. 971)—an intersection that Alondra Nelson (2011) calls a "dialectic of neglect and surveillance" (p. 164). Here we are again, just as we were in chapter two: Suspended between two or more existential poses. Prone between "state recognition of vulnerability" and "biopolitical regulation" (Oliviero, 2018, p. 248). Care-in-practice could not possibly be more contingent. Chapter four explores how some caretakers respond to such contingencies with their clients in an assistive technology clinic.

CHAPTER FOUR

Embodied Dignities in an Assistive Technology Clinic

Economic interests crisscross with scientific frameworks.
—*Eli Clare,* Brilliant Imperfection: Grappling with Cure

Although I've resisted the neoliberal urge to end my case studies on a high note, this chapter offers a bit of the "realistic hope" that Kai, a health care professional from chapter two, strived for. I earnestly believe that the last thing we need is more "sentimental scripting of hopelessness" (Bargetz, 2019, p. 185) that embodies an anthropomorphic, egoistic aversion to imagining "possibilities for being otherwise" (Grosz, 2011, p. 14). So, this chapter scales back from global health crises and end-of-life discourse to occupy a more intimate space where, I believe, it's possible to witness, up close and in real time, un/dignified care: a hospital's assistive technology clinic (hereafter, AT Clinic).[1] It's in the AT Clinic that I observed opportunities for what some scholars refer to as a "humble kind of hope" that is "rooted in ordinary practices of everyday life" (Alaimo, 2016, p. 2). Toward that end, this chapter examines the rather routine, decades-old practice of fitting wheelchair users with a new wheelchair.

First, some background. I came to this case study inspired by Jeannette Pols's (2013) ethnography of nurses' foot-washing practices and Pols's (2006) earlier work on washing patients in two psychiatric hospitals. I started to appreciate how otherwise deceptively mundane, routinized tasks—what chapter two termed "bedside in/dignities"—can have

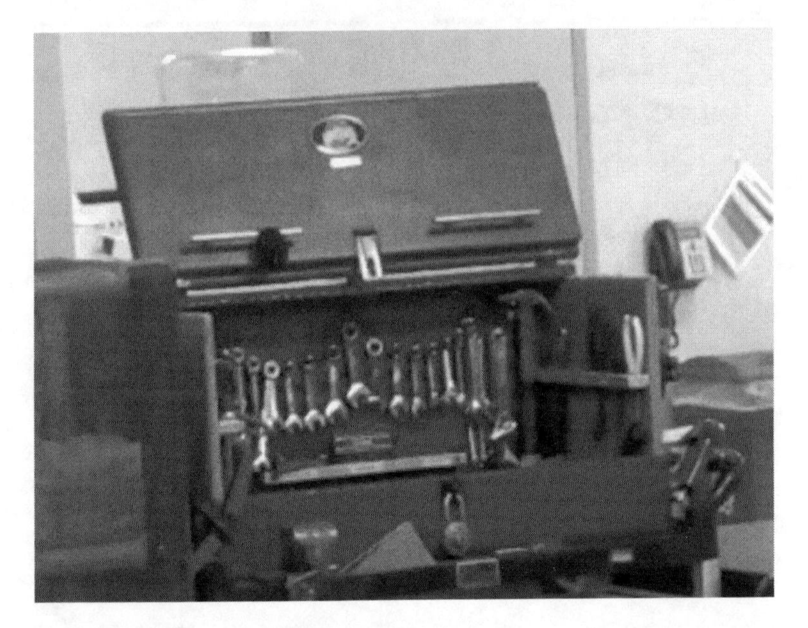

Figure 4.1. Toolbox in the center of the AT Clinic.

profound effects on human being, especially during care-in-practice, which Mol, Moser, and Pols (2015) define as "persistent tinkering in a world full of complex ambivalence and shifting tensions" (p. 14). There is perhaps no better proof that the AT Clinic is a site for tinkering than the large, bright-red toolbox that remains propped open in the center of the space (figure 4.1).

Tools from this box are continually used to tighten the bolts on a wheelchair's footrest, swap out a controller on a power wheelchair, or make tiny adjustments to the angle of a wheelchair's seat back. To this toolbox and to Mol, Moser, and Pols's "tinkering," I add the assertion that "care implies a willingness and ability *to respond*" (Brouwer & van Tuinen, 2019, p. 6; emphasis added). Responsivity manifests itself in several ways, many of which—at least in the AT Clinic—are abbreviated interactions, or what I call micro-moments. Not completely unlike the more sustained, "hard-won, organic" kind of connection Mia Mingus (2011) terms "access intimacy," micro-moments are rich with opportunities for responsivity.[2] Perpetually prone within the caretaking time-space continuum, micro-moments open up possibilities for "small, ineffable gestures that happen in everyday scenes of care" (Diedrich, 2019, p. 589). Building from chapter two's findings, I maintain that micro-moments exist "*in medias res,* in the feedback loops of transformative processes" (Brouwer and van Tuinen, p. 6). My analysis of micro-moments in the AT Clinic illustrates that doing dignity requires care workers to partner with deceptively banal, nonhuman objects, such as wheelchairs' seat cushions, as they too are important change agents that condition rhetoricity.[3]

To better understand how in/dignity emerges in clinical caretaking contexts, this chapter draws on observations of physical therapists' tactics for fitting wheelchair users for a new wheelchair. I witnessed the ways that physical therapists performed what feminist science studies calls "bodying." As a concept, bodying indexes how humans are "constitutively constrained by nature-cultural processes and relations" (Snaza, 2020, p. 182),[4] or "the body-*plus*" (Hendren, 2020, p. 29). To understand how in/dignity is (em)bodied in the AT Clinic, one must account for how care in this context is contingent on dynamic relationships between ("*Between!*" as Naomi suggested in chapter three) people, things, systems, and infrastructures.[5] As an analytic, bodying guides my interpretation of approximately 15 hours of observational data from wheelchair-fitting appointments. Bodying helps me catalogue how health care professionals—specifically, physical therapists—attempt to find a "good fit" by responding rhetorically to patients' context-dependent contingencies. Indeed, "the body is almost never not-extended" (Hendren, p. 26). Bodies result from "a dynamic relation between constraint and possibility" (Allen, 2018, p. 235). Searching for a good fit is one form of rhetorical response to bodies' contingencies.

What do I mean by "good fit"? Here, too, I'm drawing on Pols (2013): fit is a "temporary result in the process of caring" (p. 39).[6] When paired with classical rhetoric's *to prepon* ("the fitting"), fit also signifies "what is right and appropriate for the situation" (Hyde, 2006, pp. 71, 141). In the AT Clinic, as in life, fit is always conditional. Fit is an interdependent activity that is "messy, imperfect," and a constant "work-in-progress" (Clare, 2017, p. 136). Importantly, "the lack of fit," as disability studies scholars argue, "reveals the ideological assumptions controlling the space" (Siebers, 2008, p. 296). Given such messiness, I rely on systematic analyses of gestures, movement, and talk during wheelchair fitting appointments to understand how physical therapists work with clients to find a *good-enough-for-now* fit.

Without chronicling the structural conditions that produce (im)mobility in the first place—those affecting care workers whose efforts at finding a good-enough-for-now fit are frequently stymied by market-driven medicine—it's tempting to romanticize fit, especially if we perceive fit to be the "orderly and harmonious workings of nature" (Hyde, 2006, p. 71). But just like the structural conditions involved in COVID-19 caretaking described in chapter two, the AT Clinic's structural conditions require a "culture-centered approach" (Dutta, 2016, p. 17). That is, "disability cannot be abstracted from the social world which produces it; it does not exist outside the social structures in which it is located and independent of the meanings given to it" (Oliver, 1992, p. 101). Leah Lakshmi Piepzna-Samarasinha (2018) reminds us that it is "impossible to look at disability and not examine how colonialism created it" (p. 22). Although it is beyond the scope of this chapter to explicate how colonialism operates in this AT Clinic (a space that is affiliated with a land-grant institution and is, therefore, a by-product of colonial violence),[7] this chapter attempts to reconcile care-in-practice with the reality that "disability is a complex political and cultural effect of one's interaction with an environment, not simply a medical condition to be eliminated" (Dolmage & Lewiecki-Wilson, 2010, p. 30).

Numerous in/dignities at and beyond the bedside affect how fit is found in the AT Clinic. Among them is medicine's desire to normalize human bodies. For example, consider how clinics like the AT Clinic came to be. Part of the AT Clinic's biopolitical ancestry is the United Nations Rehabilitation Administration's response to "war-disability." This response resulted in legislation for rehabilitation services that would "achieve two things that seemed—on the surface—mutually compatible: (1) Reduce dependency, increase function, and help disabled soldiers reintegrate into their lives and communities. (2) Reduce the burden on society that the return of so many 'dependent' and disabled young men brought" (McPherson, Gibson, Leplège, 2015, p. 6). Just as readers witnessed the pathologizing of dependency in MAiD hearings in chapter three, the desire to normalize postwar bodies similarly pathologized dependency.

Although places like the AT Clinic now serve more than war veterans, and partnerships between rehabilitation science and disability studies continue to emerge, rehabilitation's origins affirm how intersecting biopolitical concerns about cost and vulnerability have a long legacy.

Furthermore, as we saw with how certain biopolitical topoi were operationalized in chapter three's death-with-dignity discourse, norms are propped up by "systems of inequality," including intersecting sociopolitical phenomena such as "sexism, ableism, racism, classism, heteronormativity, settler colonialism, ageism, and more" (Gupta, 2020, p. 2). Of these myriad systems of inequality, this chapter highlights how ableism, classism, and ageism intersect in ways that affect patients' experience with bodying and fit in the AT Clinic. Just because gender, race, sexuality, and colonialism do not emerge as frequently as disability, class, and age in the rest of the chapter does not mean that AT Clinic appointments were unaffected by them. Following Gupta's logic, such sociopolitical realities are always present, even if they're rendered invisible (for some researchers, myself included) "in the service of normalization" (Gupta, p. 4). Inevitably, my analyses of AT Clinic practices are constrained by (among other things) my own identity as a white, cisgender, ambulating researcher.

The following questions motivated this chapter's ethnographic observations:[8]

1. What **conditions** enable or constrain un/dignified care in the AT Clinic?
2. How do in/dignities **emerge** within (and from) human-nonhuman partnerships in the AT Clinic?
3. What does the **practice** of human dignity look like in the AT Clinic?

To investigate these three intertwined questions, I focus in particular on findings from two individuals' AT Clinic appointments (see appendix B). Through systematic analyses of field notes and transcribed video and audio data, all framed through the lens of critical disability studies and rhetorical theory, I draw readers' attention to several meaningful micro-moments that, I argue, embody what Allen (2018) describes as rhetoric's ultimate aim: living out "a kind of ethical fantasy" that might "not quite

TABLE 4.1.
AT Clinic participants and their role

Pseudonym	Role
Dean	AT Clinic patient 2
Dr. Tan	AT Clinic physician
Hazel	AT Clinic patient 1
Joe	Mobility industry vendor 1
Judy	Hazel's daughter
Loretta	Dean's daughter
Mojo	Hazel's 27-year-old wheelchair
Scott	Dean's physical therapist
Stephanie	Hazel's physical therapist
Trent	Mobility industry vendor 2

heal the world," nor does it "necessarily even make it a better place," but it "at least help(s) its subjects to be less awful at *living together in a world structured by divisions*" (p. 273; emphasis in the original).

Organization of the Chapter

First, I introduce readers to "Hazel" and her physical therapist Stephanie. Because Hazel was the individual with whom I spent the most time, the first section of my analysis draws on three of her AT Clinic appointments. Later, when I describe in greater detail the four practices I see as evidence of rhetorically responsive and dignified care, I weave in excerpts from the appointments of another individual, whom I've named "Dean." Finally, I conclude the chapter by building a localized theory about how un/dignified care can be witnessed in some of the clinic's subtler micro-moments. Before I proceed to analyzing Hazel's three appointments, I point readers to table 4.1, which lists research participants and their roles in the AT Clinic.[9]

Finding the Right Fit: Hazel's AT Clinic Appointments

At the time I began observing AT Clinic appointments in 2017, Hazel was 71 years old and had been a full-time wheelchair user for 27 years. During each of Hazel's appointments I learned more about her. Some of the earliest recordings in my field notes were of things she and I had in

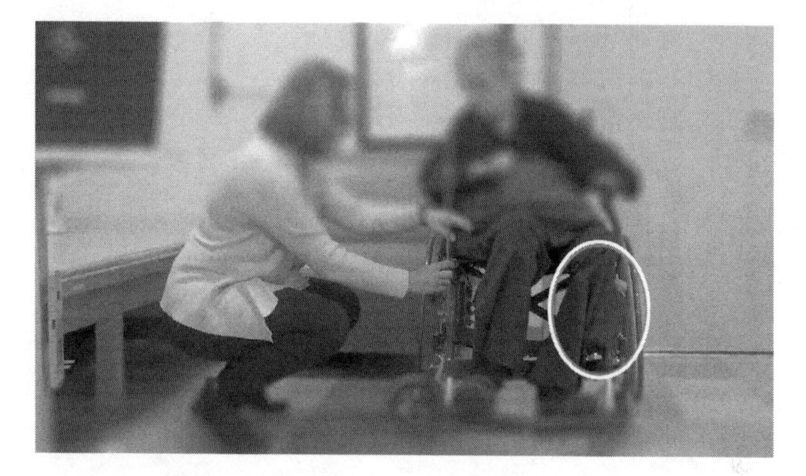

Figure 4.2. Hazel sits in her 27-year-old wheelchair, Mojo. An *oval* marks the pocket she sewed to her pants for storing items such as a water bottle.

common. We're both pianists, and we both enjoy sewing. While I'm forever trying to finish a quilt for someone, Hazel hems uniforms for her grandson's marching band. Her sewing skill is evident in how she customized her clothes. An oversized pocket holding a water bottle, conveniently attached to Hazel's left pant leg above the ankle, is one way she has made her wardrobe compatible with using a wheelchair (figure 4.2)—something Kafer (2019) might identify as "a site of crip creativity" (p. 5).

During Hazel's first two AT Clinic appointments, I also learned that she worked part-time at the local hospital. But in the last of Hazel's sessions that I observed, she appeared upset to report that she had "quit working," to which her daughter (Judy) replied, "you didn't quit mom. You retired." Hazel's (begrudged) retirement took place nearly three decades after a paralyzing motor vehicle accident in 1990. As a result of that accident, she endured a complete spinal cord injury to her fourth thoracic vertebra. Her medical record now includes paraplegia, kyphoscoliosis, and trunk instability.[10] Over time, Hazel's body adapted to her 27-year-old manual wheelchair in ways that now affect her health. Some of her concerns, which Stephanie and the AT Clinic's physician, Dr. Tan, sought to remedy with a new wheelchair, were her posture (affecting her ability to take a deep breath), pain in her back and shoulders, and pain in her legs. I also learned, when Stephanie described it to Joe, a representative of the wheelchair vendor, that Hazel relies on her elbows a lot when resituating herself in her chair. This reliance has resulted in a painful condition called ulnar entrapment.

When Dr. Tan, Stephanie, and Joe reacted with (tempered) surprise to the fact that Hazel had been using the same manual wheelchair for 27 years, she joked that it has "good mojo." At home, Hazel does, in fact, have a power wheelchair, but she reported that it just sits in a corner, unused. One reason Hazel said she does not use the power wheelchair is because its lateral support is insufficient. When Hazel answered Stephanie's questions about the power wheelchair's features, I gathered that the chair's technological affordances were outdated as well.

The other reason Hazel does not use her power wheelchair is a bit more complicated. In the first appointment, Hazel said she has "never allowed myself to use the world 'disabled' . . . so to think of a power chair, that was the first thing I thought. 'Oh no, I'm not disabled.' Of course, I am. I know I am intellectually. But I didn't . . . I don't want to feed into that yet." Hazel also told Stephanie that although she owns a wheelchair ramp designed to help her get in and out of her home, she does not want her neighbors to see it. Hazel's fraught relationship with her disability (and impending retirement) may explain Stephanie's approach at the start of the first appointment: "Dr. Tan and I both have medical recommendations for things that you don't want. So, what I was talking to the vendor about earlier today was . . . We talked about a power wheelchair and what those would do. But we are both respectful. That's your body. And you have a certain lifestyle. And we're going to do the best we can to meet your goals." An especially skilled physical therapist and, I would argue, rhetorician, Stephanie spent most of the appointment trying to reconcile Hazel's preferences, feelings, and experiences with standardized medical expertise and recommendations. The primary fit-related conundrum that Hazel and her care team appeared to be working through is Hazel's reluctance to adopt a new power wheelchair—a reluctance that persists despite all the ways her 27-year-old manual wheelchair may be doing her more harm than good.

Before discussing pain, ability, or even cost, Stephanie starts the appointment by reiterating to Hazel that she, Dr. Tan, and Joe are all going to "give you our opinions," but "at no time" are they "trying to disrespect you or push you in any direction that you don't feel comfortable."

> STEPHANIE: When we talk about a power wheelchair . . . I can only imagine how that has to do *THIS* [hits chest with closed fist] to you.
> HAZEL: Oh yeah, it does.
> STEPHANIE: Yeah, and so that's . . . I just . . . I bridge that cautiously.

When transcribing this exchange, I found no referent for the word "*THIS*." I imagine sociolinguists probably have a word for phenomena like it, but in any case, Hazel and Stephanie played along as though they shared an understanding of what *THIS* was. Although its specifics were never stated during the appointment, I see it as evidence of Stephanie's empathy for Hazel's situation. As I discussed in chapter one, though, *THIS* is fleeting. *THIS*, along with the thump of Stephanie's closed fist on her chest, embodies rhetoric's "nonhermeneutic, ethical" dimension (Davis, 2010, p. 69). Its contours unspool as the appointment moves toward a more medicalized discussion of Hazel's situation.

Hazel's posture contributes to her pain. But her pain also contributes to her posture. Specifically, Hazel's posture is the result of her abdominal muscles having weakened over time and of her wheelchair's incapacity to hold her upright. One of the goals for the appointment, therefore, was to try out assistive technologies,[11] such as custom back support, that would help Hazel sit up straighter. Combined with wearing an abdominal binder, a new wheelchair with custom back support would (medically) improve Hazel's posture. Such interventions may not just alleviate some of Hazel's pain, but they may also let her take deeper breaths. And for disabilities like Hazel's, having the capacity to breathe deeply is key. In fact, at the time I conducted my observations at the AT Clinic, the United States was in the throes of an awful influenza season. And as I write this chapter, the world is facing off with variant after variant of COVID-19. If Hazel were to contract a respiratory infection, it could settle in her lungs and develop into a life-threatening disease. It's not an understatement to say that Hazel's survival could hinge on assistive technology.

In addition to their implicit goal of survival is Hazel and Stephanie's more explicit desire to alleviate musculoskeletal pain. When reciting a rationale that Joe might include in his justification to Hazel's insurance company, Stephanie hypothesized that Hazel wasn't using her existing power chair because it's "pretty big and bulky. Am I right?" Hazel hesitated in saying yes and then added some quite meaningful details:

HAZEL: What is it, too, is uhh. [tone grows more animated, begins to gesture with right hand] When I'm up and moving around, regardless of what I feel . . . the circulation is better [gestures with right hand in a circle motion close to right leg]. So, by the end of the day [points down], after work [points thumb behind her], I'm better! [gives thumbs-up gesture] So, I'm thinking: If I'm in a power chair [points toward Stephanie], I'm not using my arms [gestures toward self]. I'm not using the circulation. [makes circular gesture in air] I don't feel as good! And I don't do as much at home! [rests hands on lap, turns to look at Joe] I do very little! [smiles]

STEPHANIE: Mmhmm.

HAZEL: So I think, yeah. [in a more solemn, quieter tone] But the posture of course is the top priority. [near whisper] With the scoliosis. [shrugs and looks off to the side]

Hazel's verbal and nonverbal rationale in this exchange that lasted no more than 30 seconds suggests to me that her resistance to a power chair is rooted in a concern that, without the physical exertion presently required to operate her manual wheelchair, her body will decline for lack of exercise.

By the end of this micro-moment, when Hazel's affect appears to shift as she concedes that "posture is a top priority," I hear evidence of what Jacobson (2012) might identify as the beginnings of a "dignity bargain." When someone makes a "dignity bargain," she "gives up some dignity to get something else she needs" (p. 153). In the exchange above, Hazel seems to relinquish hope that she will be able to maintain physical fitness by continuing to use a manual wheelchair. The trade-off, were she to adopt a power wheelchair, is that her posture will likely change in ways that alleviate pain and improve pulmonary function. As Hazel considers such a bargain, Stephanie recognizes the rhetorical challenge. Stephanie must find a way to make this trade-off less of a violation to

Hazel's sense of self. This is a tall order, since the very technology of a power wheelchair poses a kind of embodied threat to Hazel.

In the passage below, Hazel recounts what happened at her last appointment when she trialed a new power wheelchair:

> HAZEL: And I would push [makes circular gesture with index fingers of both hands] and then it would put me around [makes gripping gesture with both hands]. I lost control! [rests both hands on lap, raises eyebrows, and shakes head back and forth]
>
> STEPHANIE: That's right. And so the thing that we were talking about was that the . . . the sensitivity with your balance, you couldn't get an equal stroke.
>
> HAZEL: Right.

So, in addition to her concern about not getting enough physical exertion, Hazel's frightening experience previously with one power wheelchair seems to have biased her against a power wheelchair, despite Stephanie's and Dr. Tan's medically sound recommendations. Nevertheless, Stephanie continued to work with Joe to find a sophisticated enough power (or power-assist) wheelchair to accommodate Hazel's preferred propelling habits—embodied tactics that have been shaped by nearly three decades of manual wheelchair use.

The handful of meaningful micro-moments I've described thus far come from just the first 15 minutes of Hazel's first AT Clinic appointment.[12] Such moments are rich with important information about how Hazel's im/mobility is conditioned. Below, I provide a bird's-eye view of six significant events that occurred during the whole of the first appointment. Note that things got tense between events 3 and 4 when Hazel appeared frustrated while trialing power-assist wheelchairs:

1. Stephanie summarizes for Hazel some of Dr. Tan's notes and emphasizes, through verbal reasoning and explicit recognition of Hazel's unique experiences, that she and Joe are there to meet Hazel's goals and priorities.
2. Through a series of simulations, Hazel "plays with" one power-assist wheelchair (chair A) while Stephanie compares the differences between chair A and Hazel's current manual wheelchair (Mojo).

Hazel trials chair A on a ramp that is built to standards of the Americans with Disabilities Act and on another ramp that is not. Hazel also trials the chair on the clinic's other sloped surfaces.[13]

3. Hazel doesn't appear to like chair A. So Stephanie shows Hazel a different power-assist chair (chair B) while describing how it compares with both chair A and Mojo. Stephanie herself trials chair B on the clinic's ramps and slopes.
4. Stephanie invites Hazel to play with chair B. Hazel declines to try it and transfers from chair A back to Mojo.
5. Stephanie pivots away from medicalized reasoning to accommodate Hazel's preferences and concerns.
6. By the end of the two-hour appointment, Hazel and Stephanie settle on a new manual wheelchair (chair C) rather than a power-assist or full-power chair.

Because of how fraught the appointment became between events 3 and 4, I am missing an entire hour of video data, as I made the decision to stop recording. I could sense that Stephanie and Joe were working hard to reconcile Hazel's preferences with their medicalized recommendations. Worried that following them around with a video camera could hinder a resolution, I opted to rely instead on my memory and field notes.

Hazel's second AT Clinic appointment involved finding the right fit through a host of iterative measurements of, and modifications to, chair C. Stephanie also showed Hazel therapeutic movements she could practice at home to alleviate pain. Importantly, Stephanie described how these movements would affect Hazel's anatomy, and she did so in a way that was intelligible to listeners who lacked medical knowledge of the human body.

The third AT Clinic appointment was scheduled on a whim just after Hazel received chair C and wanted to discuss with Stephanie some of the (expected) fit-related issues she was experiencing. During this appointment, Stephanie showed Hazel how to put pressure on her funny bone to relieve pain caused by ulnar entrapment. At one point, Stephanie had everyone huddle around her laptop to watch a YouTube video demonstrating how to perform a therapeutic movement called the "Tyler Twist."

Thus far, I have provided both a fine-grained selection and an enumerated summary of Hazel's AT Clinic appointments. Now that readers have a sense of who and what were involved in a typical AT Clinic appointment, I describe how all the AT Clinic appointments unfolded—including how "contingency" emerged as an important finding in my analysis.[14]

Fit-Related Activities and Actors in the AT Clinic

Early observations of AT Clinic appointments yielded a long list of activities and actors.[15] In particular, Level 1 activities were those that any sighted researcher could observe during an appointment. These included things like writing, listening, and kneeling. Level 2 activities required some inference-making about what was going on. For example, "reasoning" was the discursive marker I used as shorthand for several co-constitutive activities, such as considering cost versus benefit, watching how a patient responds to a particular wheelchair, and perhaps even mentioning a patient's preferred hobbies. Activity levels allowed me to document how atomized Level 1 activities developed into more meaningful practices. The actors listed in box 4.1 range from the particular (e.g., transfer board) to the general (e.g., wheelchairs).

After repeatedly comparing the activities and actors catalogued in box 4.1, I rewatched all of my AT Clinic video recordings and noted that several activities and actors would coalesce around or co-constitute one another in ways that led to larger, more complex phenomena. I had not accounted for these yet because my analyses up to that point had been so fine-grained. These phenomena are what I decided to call a "contingency."

A contingency might involve one or more Level 2 activities and several actors, for example. Contingencies, in the context of this case study, are micro-moments during AT Clinic appointments when it was clear that a decision about fit needed to be made, the options for which were neither straightforward nor perfect, and yet *not* responding risked ushering in a worse (or at least undesirable) outcome. As Hyde (2006) reminds us, "there always comes uncertainty and contingency with the openness of Being" (p. 67). In the AT Clinic, I see finding a good fit, or bodying, as quintessential "openness of Being."

A prime example of contingency is Hazel's worry that, without the exertion required to operate a manual wheelchair, her body would stiffen,

BOX 4.1.

Activities and actors in Hazel's AT Clinic appointments

Level 1 activities

writing / typing / moving / listening / watching / supporting / touching / transferring / kneeling / assembling / modifying / rolling / walking / talking / gesturing / reading

Level 2 activities

considering / claiming / reasoning / assisting / demonstrating / simulating / comparing / affirming / testing / measuring / teaching / introducing / summarizing / reviewing

Actors

wheelchairs / insurance companies / people / tools / clinic space / vehicles or transportation / time / internet / furniture / past experience / laptops / mobile desks / tables / wheels / cushions / wheelchair backs / straps / YouTube / extant research / popularized physical therapy / headrests / chairs (standard and extra wide) / legs / elbows / feet / chin / hands / arms / abdomen / shoulders / back / duct tape / footrest / ramp / slope / mirror / scale / laptop sticker / bulletin boards / printouts / markers on floor (red tape) / hallway / iPhone / toolbox / wrench set / wheels / writing technologies / stool / anti-tippers / motor / battery pack / common area / private room / transfer board / measuring stick / physical therapists / vendors / doctors / clients / family members / support staff / documents

she wouldn't feel as good, and her health would decline. Contingency in this case marks a moment when Hazel reasons (a Level 2 activity) based on her past experiences (as an actor) with how her body feels before and after certain kinds of movements. As she described this worry—a moment of "openness of Being"—she relied on a host of communicative tactics, including gestures and other forms of embodied communication. Contingencies were important to document, as they forced me to recognize how others *responded* to said contingencies. I argue that it is in care workers' responses to a *contingency* that one witnesses possibilities for un/dignified care. Notably, un/dignified care is not always correlated with discursive markers that index empathy or a shared experience (such as "*THIS*" described earlier in the chapter).

The contingencies I encountered in the AT Clinic across every patient's appointment exemplify what Astrida Neimanis (2017) describes as "the paradox of bodies":

> Thus, the paradox of bodies—bodies that we are willing to defend to the death, even as we know they are falling apart at the seams—is not, as Elizabeth Grosz would say, a problem to be solved. Most big problems, Grosz (2012: 14) reminds us, "like the problem of gravity, of living with others, or that of mortality, have no solutions"; instead we need to seek "ways of living with problems." In other words, the challenge is not to solve the feminist paradox of bodies, but rather to experiment in how to live this paradox, and live it well. (p. 18)

The contingency code that developed from AT Clinic micro-moments accounts for problems that "have no solutions"—emergent phenomena that require physical therapists and their clients to negotiate "ways of living with problems" (Neimanis, p. 18). Stephanie and Hazel responded to contingencies by negotiating a way to *live* (well and) *with* the inevitability of corporeal change, *in medias res,* even if that change results in increased stiffness.[16]

For all participants in this study, numerous contingencies emerged that affected fit. As a reminder, fit was about more than a wheelchair's physical specifications. In addition to physical specifications and technological affordances, fit was also informed by the following contingencies (to name just a few):

- a patient's relationship with their own disability;
- the possibility of new diagnoses and corporeal experiences affecting pain and perceived exertion;

- the degree to which insurance companies will cover specific options;
- the type of vehicle the patient will use to transport their wheelchair; and
- what's available for trialing at the clinic (e.g., some demo chairs have dead batteries or broken wheels).

Care workers' attempts at responding to the contingencies described above exemplify what Davis (2010) might characterize as obligatory moments of addressivity—the real-time response to an Other's "exposure to exposedness" (p. 11). When I refer to "exposure to exposedness," I am drawing most immediately on Davis's work. But, ultimately, Davis is invoking continental philosophers (e.g., Jean Luc Nancy and Levinas) to highlight what I interpret instead as a more fine-grained account of stratified livability (Manderson, Burke, & Wahlberg, 2021) and varying vulnerability (Niccolini & Ringrose, 2019), which hinges on a precise moment in time wherein an Other's vulnerability is recognized and potentially acknowledged.[17] Importantly, during an "exposure to exposedness" encounter, "nonresponse is not an option" (Davis p. 12). Episodes of exposedness, as Mbembe (2019) describes, enable "a *relation of care*" (p. 176; emphasis in the original). Episodes of exposedness aren't always spectacular, either. They're often quite mundane, in fact.

I see options for responding to an Other's exposedness as existing on a rhetorical continuum, where full-on acknowledgment anchors one end and mere recognition the other (more on that to come in the next chapter). Recall from chapter one that acknowledgment "is an act whereby we open ourselves to things and to others in order to foster and maintain a close (loving) relationship with them" (Hyde, 2006, p. 53). Likening it to a Levinasian "caress," Hyde describes how "acknowledgment and the caress . . . work together to accomplish the ethical task of home-making" (p. 117). For the purpose of this chapter, think of "home-making" as the practice of wheelchair fitting. In the micro-moments I describe in the next section, I highlight where Hazel's and Dean's exposedness became evident and how other actors in the clinic responded to that exposedness. To make exposedness more detectable, and inspired by Ellingson's (2017) work on accounting for embodiment in qualitative research,[18] I include

BOX 4.2.

Activities in response to AT Clinic contingencies

simulating / comparing / verbal reasoning / recognizing / showing / teaching / measuring / modifying

verbal descriptions of participants' gestures as they negotiated fit-related contingencies. AT Clinic actors responded rhetorically through the eight mundane activities listed in box 4.2.[19]

Specifically, it was when I witnessed *pairings* of these eight activities that the conditions for dignified care seemed to emerge. Ultimately, I see four pairs of activities as practices that embody dignified care in the AT Clinic:

— Practice 1: simulate+compare
— Practice 2: reason+recognize
— Practice 3: show+teach
— Practice 4: measure+modify

Four Practices That Embody Dignified Care in the AT Clinic

There is nothing inherently dignified about any of the activities listed in box 4.2. Rather, when physical therapists creatively paired particular activities, I detected a notable shift in how a contingency was addressed. That shift may have involved a patient divulging a private concern, for example. The shift might also have been signaled by an abundance of positive affect that seemed apparent to everyone in the room. When *simulating* was paired with *comparing*, *reasoning* with *recognizing*, *showing* with *teaching*, and *measuring* with *modifying*, conditions for dignified care were evident. It is impossible, of course, to infer a causal link between these four practices and human dignity. Since mine is a descriptive study that relies on interpretivist methods, I can only assert that these four

TABLE 4.2.
Practices that create conditions for dignified care in the AT Clinic

Practice	Definition
Simulate+Compare	Experientially "playing with" an assistive technology in the AT Clinic's artificially designed contexts, while verbally comparing said experiences with previous and/or future mobility experiences
Reason+Recognize	Leveraging a well-supported claim about fit that is accompanied by validation of another's experiences, needs, and desires
Show+Teach	Materially and verbally demonstrating features and affordances of a potential solution in a way that is intelligible to someone without discipline-specific (e.g., engineering, biomechanical, biomedical) expertise
Measure+Modify	Assessing fit by employing a measuring tool of some kind and, based on measurements taken, making material changes to an assistive technology to improve fit

practices in this AT Clinic seeded conditions for dignified care to emerge. In table 4.2, I identify and define the four practices.[20]

Each of these four practices helped to facilitate fit by responding rhetorically to a contingency. That is, such practices created a space wherein AT Clinic participants could

- collaboratively assess the effects that certain material configurations might have on a future outcome;
- communicate about anticipated barriers and changes; and
- consider heretofore unanticipated external influences (e.g., undignified asides).

The remainder of this chapter is devoted to describing these four practices in detail, as witnessed during AT Clinic appointments with Hazel and with another individual, Dean.

Practice 1: Simulate+Compare

The first practice includes two activities one might expect to see in the AT Clinic: Hazel and Dean simulate within the built space of the clinic what it's like to use a particular wheelchair, while Stephanie and Scott prompt Hazel and Dean to compare the effects of a simulated fit with previous or anticipated experiences. As figure 4.3 shows, the clinic space

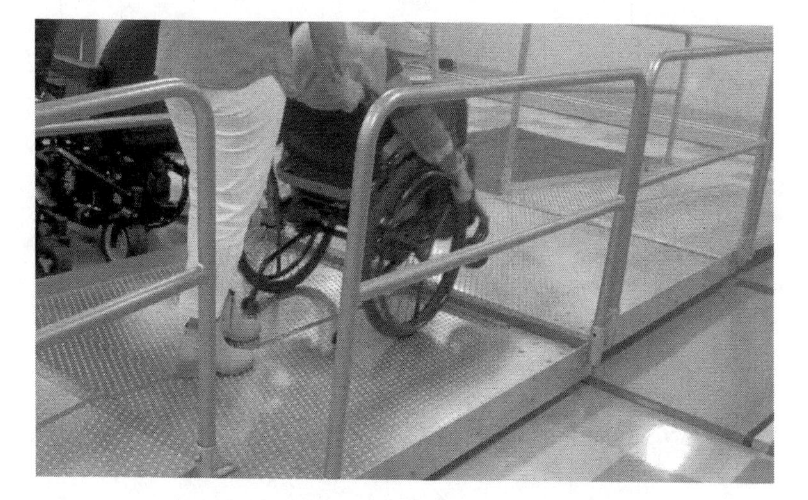

Figure 4.3. The AT Clinic's ramp, which includes a seven-degree grade for simulating wheelchair experiences. With Stephanie behind her, Hazel is performing a "wheelie" in chair A to maneuver over a two-inch-high ridge in the ramp.

contains a ramp with a seven-degree grade as well as several other slopes designed to simulate what it's like to operate a wheelchair on surfaces that are built to code versus those not built to code. Although the AT Clinic cannot anticipate all the ways the built world neglects disabled persons' mobility experiences, the clinic's inclusion of a variety of mobility barriers—for instance, slopes with a steep grade, uneven surfaces, ramps with either smooth or textured surfaces—facilitate opportunities for Hazel and Dean to make decisions about fit during simulation activities.[21]

As Hazel and Dean practiced simulations with various wheelchairs (and fits), physical therapists either offered or invited feedback about how a simulated experience compared with current or past mobility experiences, especially as those experiences related to a (quantifiable) sense of pain and rating of perceived exertion.[22] Here's Mol (2021): "The *doing* staged in this way is not confined to a moment—of choice—nor is it linear—like a causal chain. Instead, it is of a caring—iterative, adaptive, tinkering—kind" (p. 86). So, when Stephanie and Scott held space for Hazel's and Dean's reflections on how the fit experienced during the simulation compared with their previous fit-related experiences, more nuanced discussions emerged of how the wheelchair could be adapted or tinkered with to achieve a "less dissatisfying" fit (Allen, 2018, p. 275). Often, the simulate+compare practice acted as a prelude to practices of reason+recognize and measure+modify.

Practice 2: Reason+Recognize

When reasoning verbally about fit, participants invoked several forms of evidence, including, for example,

- financial costs associated with a wheelchair's distinct design;
- nuances of a wheelchair's technical specifications; and
- potential benefits of a wheelchair's unique features.

On its own, though, verbal reasoning could take discussions about fit only so far. When paired with recognition, verbal reasoning seemed to become supercharged. That is, verbal reasoning, when paired meaningfully with Stephanie's and Scott's explicit recognition of Hazel's and Dean's unique experiences, needs, and desires, responded to a contingency more directly. Let me provide an example.

In the exchange below, Scott and Loretta (Dean's daughter) begin Dean's appointment by updating Trent (the wheelchair vendor) about what kind of wheelchair would be a good fit for Dean as his Parkinson's disease continued to advance. In the background of this exchange is the fact that the wheelchairs equipped with the features Dean needs aren't built for his body weight—what I would characterize as an "undignified aside."

SCOTT: [seated across from Dean and Loretta, reading from laptop screen] Dr. Tan and I feel like Dean needs a group three power wheelchair with tilt and elevating [indiscernible]. And we also talked about power seat elevator [gestures right hand upward toward ceiling] and even anterior tilt a little bit [gestures right hand downward toward the ground].

[Scott turns head to look at Trent]

SCOTT: Just as, like, ways that he could be more independent.

[Scott turns head back to look at Dean]

SCOTT: Power seat elevator would be really good because it would allow you to be up higher when you're in crowds.

LORETTA: His anxiety, yes.

SCOTT: Yeah, because there are times when you get anxious when you're in large groups of people [gestures both hands up toward ceiling, pace of speaking increases] and they can't see you and you feel like you can't see. So, you get nervous. [looks back at laptop screen]

DEAN: I went to the Ohio State Fair last year. So. Yeah.

Here, Scott recognizes and honors Dean's anxiety about being low to the ground in his wheelchair while stuck in crowds. Dean, in turn, alludes to a vulnerable, potentially traumatic experience at the state fair. The remainder of the appointment, then, is geared toward finding a fit that would enable Dean to feel less anxious and better supported in crowded situations. Along the way, however, the proverbial elephant in the room—the undignified aside—is the fact that wheelchair manufacturers fail to account fully for variations in human bodies' shapes and sizes. This will have a negative effect on Dean's care, no matter how hard Scott works to fine-tune fit.

Note how, in the next exchange below, wheelchair vendor Trent tries to navigate the constraint created by wheelchair manufacturers, who are, at best, unaccountable to varying vulnerability and are, at worst, fat-phobic. In this moment, Trent (awkwardly) tries to respond to the same contingency described above but in a way that pits Dean's non-normative body weight against his mobility options.

TRENT: [seated across from Dean at mobile desk, behind laptop, looking at Loretta, and fidgeting with both hands under desk] No, I mean, you know, anterior tilt is also going to fall under that equation. Sometimes there's one brand that does a little bit more of it. [scratches left knee] I feel like the Permobile . . . But the one thing we'll have to look at, too, is I think . . . with our weight over the three hundred (pound) mark . . . is some of those anterior options aren't . . . [gestures right hand up above laptop] There was some ten degree . . . [kicks left leg out and rests left hand on left knee] There were some small anterior tilts that came with the seat elevators [pushes desk away from body by a few inches, scratches knee again]. But I think because we're over a certain [weight] threshold, they may not have the same options for that [brings both hands back under desk and begins fidgeting again].

LORETTA: Ok.

TRENT: So just, you know [shrugs], just a little bit of a wild card thing. Just, we have to consider . . .

LORETTA: [interrupting] Which outweighs?

TRENT: Which is more important? Like, the seat . . .

LORETTA: [interrupting] Correct.

TRENT: The seat. I mean I think the seat elevate seems to be. Yeah, that's probably . . .

SCOTT: I would think so. The anterior tilt we talked about last time because of his . . . [Loretta interrupts while Scott gestures with right hand, elbow resting on desk, pinky pointing toward Dean]

LORETTA: [interrupting] Pressure. His tailbone. [removes purse from around body and places it on floor]

SCOTT: His chair currently . . . He has like a lift chair? [looks at Loretta]

LORETTA: [leans back up after placing purse on floor] Correct.

SCOTT: And that's one of the only ways he's able to get up consistently [looks over at Trent] especially when he's tired and he's having, you know, more problems with akinesia.

Note that Dean is verbally absent (or silenced) in the exchange above. I'll also add that Trent's shift toward stand-alone reasoning (sans recognition) ushers in one of only a handful of moments during the appointment when Scott talks *about* Dean instead of *to* Dean.

It's likely that because Trent's presence in this exchange is guided by his sales role, he's inclined to rely more on the technical specifications in reasoning how certain chairs would be a good fit. It's a subtle shift, but Trent's stand-alone verbal reasoning precipitates what I regard as a potentially dehumanizing experience for Dean, who watches while others talk *about* rather than *to* him and allude to his weight (which Trent patronizingly calls "our weight"). Dean watches while others interject priorities without leaving space for him to contribute to the conversation. In fact, the only thing we hear from Dean during this exchange is the sound of his tremoring hand on the fabric pouch that holds additional medical supplies. Perhaps coincidentally, the sound of Dean's "demi-rhetorical" tremor on the fabric pouch gets louder as the above exchange continues without him (Yergeau, 2018, p. 179).[23]

The bridge that connects the two moments described above is the exchange below wherein another fit-related contingency emerges, this time concerning finances:

> SCOTT: Ok. We did talk last time about funding challenges with some of those things. How Medicare just traditionally has not covered that feature [smiles at Dean, shakes head]. No matter what we do.
>
> LORETTA: Yeah.
>
> SCOTT: How long have we fought? [looks at Dean] They just don't . . . but it may be an option that you could pay for or figure out some way [looks at Trent] we could get some of the funding for that [looks at Loretta].

It may be a coincidence that financial constraints—yet more undignified asides—precipitated the stand-alone verbal reasoning that Trent engages in above. Nevertheless, I think it's important to note that economic concerns are flanked by two types of responses to Dean's exposedness. The latter attempt relied on verbal reasoning alone, while the former (with its talk of Dean's seat height) relied on verbal reasoning and recognition of Dean's experiences. Pairing reasoning with recognition seemed to create the conditions for dignified care to emerge, whereas stand-alone reasoning was potentially dehumanizing for Dean. One might refer to these two approaches as a "battle of cares," where, in Dean's case, the practice of pairing reason with recognition became "an antidote to the instrumental life that the systems of the market and governance demand we live" (Klamer, 2019, p. 188).

Practice 3: Show+Teach

Approximately 20 minutes into Hazel's first appointment, as she and Stephanie discussed the need for a wheelchair that has custom back support, Stephanie used an abdominal binder and a pop can analogy to show and then teach Hazel about how to supplement core strength while living with a spinal cord injury. Here is the exchange:

STEPHANIE: One of the best comparisons I've ever heard for spinal cord injury is a pop can. So, think of a Pepsi when the top tab and all that pressure is closed, it's got a lot of solid control through the core. So, comparing the pop can to your trunk, okay? [gestures with both hands up and down her waist] And as soon as that pop can is open [gestures to imitate opening a pop can], that pop can can just be crushed [gestures to imitate crushing a can]. So that stability, that internal pressure that's coming is like our muscular support. And when you don't have that, your body just crumbles [slumps shoulders down and leans back, to imitate crumbling]. And so, to gain some of that back, a binder [overlaps both hands over lower abdomen], or something that draws you into a contoured back support [exaggerates pulling shoulders back and down the spine], can help give some of that pressure, control, stability.

[Hazel nods]

STEPHANIE: And so, for some of my clients, we've made custom backs . . . with Velcro buckle that you buckle it in place [gestures to imitate buckling a belt around waist]. If you don't use it, you swing it to the back of you [swings both hands behind back].

HAZEL: Like a corset . . .

JOE: Mmhmm.

STEPHANIE: Yeah. So, when the chair has a little bit of this downward slope, so that gravity [gestures down], and it helps pull you up, and then you can lean into that back support [exaggerates pulling shoulders back and down the spine]. And the good thing is with your body shape is that you're not a round or a square, you have shape to you [gestures the shape of an hourglass]. And so, the good thing with the custom back is that it can hold on to your rib cage, when you've got that women's shape to you.

[Hazel nods]

STEPHANIE: So, I think that you're a good candidate, as long as it doesn't restrict you from activity too much.

HAZEL: Yes.

STEPHANIE: Because right now, if you wanted to pick something up off the floor [points toward ground] . . .

HAZEL: [looks to side of wheelchair and tries to bend at the waist while wearing the abdominal binder] Probably can't.

STEPHANIE: Probably can't.

HAZEL: And you don't want to always have to carry around one of those little uhh . . .

STEPHANIE: Yeah, you got it. And then the other thing is, is pretend this is your piano, right? [gestures to the left of Hazel]

HAZEL: It would be. Yeah. Well, I don't think I can get under a piano anyway. So, I . . . because it's not . . . it's too short. So, I would go from the side to play the piano.

STEPHANIE: But the thing is, is that [points to abdominal binder] still limits how far you can twist this [points to waist] to get to it [gestures a twisting motion].

HAZEL: Oh, ok yeah.

STEPHANIE: It's just a consideration with the piano. Playing a keyboard [gestures to opposite side of Hazel] is not the same as playing piano [gestures back toward the imaginary piano].

[Hazel nods]

STEPHANIE: Yeah, so some people but some people have said, "Well, I'll just change to a keyboard."

HAZEL: But it's an option. You know, I thought about it.

STEPHANIE: I play the piano [touches chest]. It's not the same, like, you know, exactly.

[Everyone laughs; Hazel nods excitedly]

STEPHANIE: It's not the same! Exactly! I like that pressure piano key sound.

In this exchange between Hazel and Stephanie, Stephanie is gesturally showing and teaching Hazel about the corporeal effect an abdominal binder will have on supporting her core, which, as I described earlier, is a necessary response to Hazel's exposedness given how important core support is for being able to breathe and cough. At the same time, she's also engaging in verbal reasoning accompanied by recognition of Hazel's piano playing.[24] This episode illustrates how Stephanie and Hazel collaborated to find the right fit and, in response to several contingencies, Stephanie paired showing and teaching as well as reasoning and recognition. The enthusiasm I witnessed in Hazel's nonverbal responses to Stephanie's gestures about piano playing marked an energy shift in the room. The trepidation that Hazel may have had about the appointment, given her reluctance to transition to a power wheelchair, seemed to disappear momentarily. However short-lived that moment of relief was, it happened; and it embodied what I saw as an example of dignified care.

During Dean's appointment, his daughter, Loretta, worried about Dean's capacity to control his own chair as his disease advances. Currently, Dean relied on a mobility scooter that was insufficient for his needs. At the start of Dean's first simulation experience in the new power wheelchair, Dean wheeled off toward the ramp, and Loretta exclaimed, "Oh gosh! Giving him independence! Ahhh!" Prior to Loretta's expression of nervous reluctance, much earlier in the appointment, Loretta had asked Scott about installing "attendant control" on Dean's new power wheelchair. Attendant controls are typically mounted behind the wheelchair user so that someone behind them can control the chair's functionality. Recognizing how that might affect Dean's sense of independence and agency, Scott tactfully nipped that in the bud.

SCOTT: [looking at Loretta] But remember you can always drive the chair just standing next to it with Dean's joystick.

LORETTA: Mmhmm.

SCOTT: You know what I mean? You don't have to have another controller . . .

LORETTA: Right.

SCOTT: . . . on the back of the chair to drive it. You can just stand next to it and drive, which is what actually I [gestures toward self] prefer to do.

LORETTA: Ok.

SCOTT: Because I think it's easier for me to do that. But . . .

LORETTA: [interrupting] Scooter-wise it was hard. [laughs]

SCOTT: Oh, yeah, nearly impossible! [gestures arms as if they're wrapping around a large object]

LORETTA: [laughing] Yeah.

SCOTT: 'Cause you'd have to get on [motions arms together as if trying to reach around a large object] . . .

LORETTA: [laughing awkwardly] Yeah.

SCOTT: So, it's something to think about. . . .

LORETTA: [interrupting] And then oxygen for his . . .

SCOTT: Yeah, oxygen too. [looks down at laptop and clicks button on mouse, turns toward Trent] So I think the best thing to do now, Trent, is just grab . . . we have the M300 [model], right?

In this exchange Scott makes it as clear as he can to Loretta that the forthcoming process of finding a good fit for Dean, even while responding to a host of personalized contingencies, does not require that Dean sacrifice his own independence or control. As disability studies scholars clarify, "the ability to *act as a self* remains a contested life-or-death issue for many people with disabilities—especially those who are multiply marginalized by race, gender, sexuality, age, and/or class" (Belser, 2016, 14; emphasis in the original). This moment in Dean's appointment doesn't represent the show+teach practice; rather it demonstrates how powerful show+teach was as a practice throughout the *rest* of Dean's appointment. Fifty-two of the 63 minutes in Dean's appointment involved a series of show+teach practices where Dean was both shown and taught (verbally, with accessible directives) how to operate a new power wheelchair. Even though Loretta requested "attendant control" so that she could control her dad's wheelchair, Scott spent most of the appointment showing+teaching Dean how to manage his own mobility.

Later, when Scott was showing Dean where certain buttons were on his chair (figure 4.4), the following exchange took place:

[Dean presses a button on his chair, which makes a beep sound]

SCOTT: That's the power. And you can use these buttons here [points at buttons on Dean's chair, looks at Dean]. They're like shortcut keys for the power features. The one that you're going to have or one of the ones you're going to have is this one here. The tilt. And also the elevator. This one is recline. You won't have this one yet in your chair because you don't really need this one yet as far as your medical problems go. And then this one's the power seat elevator we talked about.

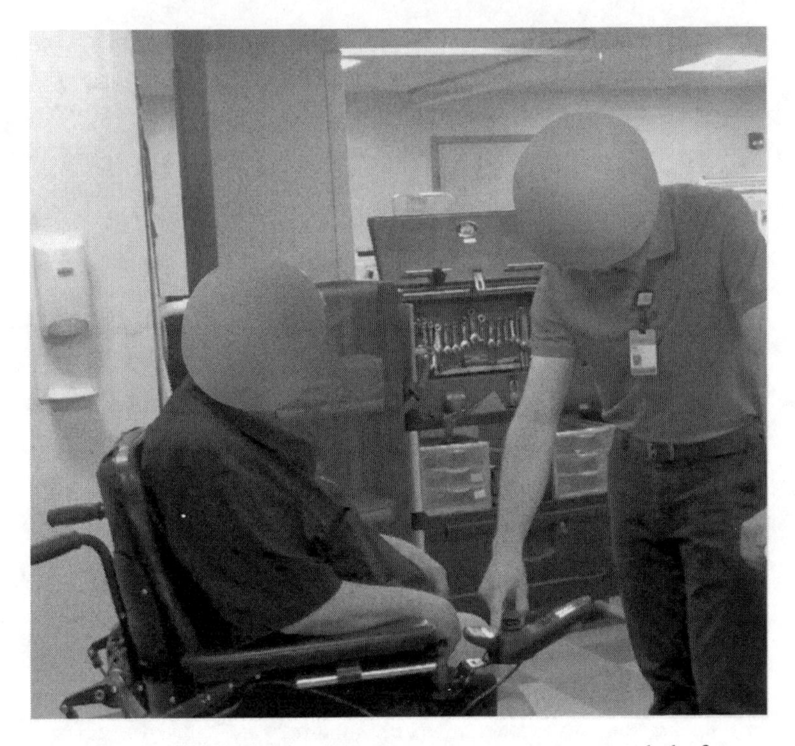

Figure 4.4. In an instance of show+teach, Scott acquaints Dean with the features of a demo wheelchair.

DEAN: Different size . . . like for the coffee table and the restaurant?

SCOTT: Yeah! [stands upright and takes a step back away from Dean's chair] Check that one out. Go ahead, hit the "up" key there.

[Dean presses the key; seat slowly raises]

Here, Scott both shows and teaches Dean how to operate the seat-elevate feature. This moment is important not just because it exemplifies the show+teach practice but also because it responds to one of the contingencies expressed earlier in Dean's appointment: his desire, based on past experiences, to be at eye level with people instead of sitting low to the ground. Figure 4.5 shows Scott, mid-gesture, when he excitedly said to Dean, "you can see now! Instead of you looking up at people, right? You're now eye level, right?! If there was a countertop or high-top table, you could probably sit at it without a problem, right?! You could reach

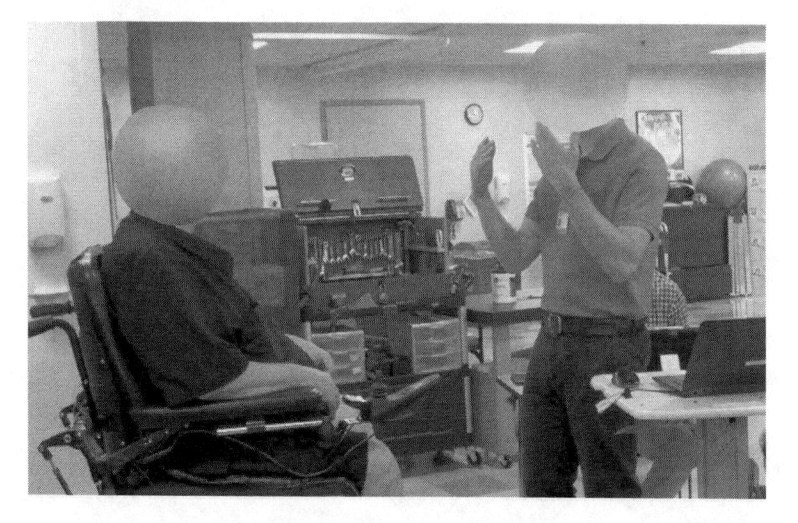

Figure 4.5. In another instance of show+teach, Scott explains to Dean the power wheelchair's seat-elevate feature, which addresses Dean's anxiety about sitting low in crowds.

into cabinets that were higher up!" Dean nods continually in response to Scott's excited queries and then responds with a joke: "Won't be able to ask the kids anymore, 'Can you get that?'" Scott and Dean share a brief laugh and continue with more show+teach moments.

Practice 4: Measure+Modify

Finally, the act of measuring includes a range of activities, like documenting distances between two or more points (e.g., knee to footrest), using pressure-mapping technology to visualize whether a patient's buttocks rest on a wheelchair's seat cushion in a way that risks pressure sores, and counting the number of pushes it takes for a patient to roll from one place to another (figure 4.6).

When measuring was combined with modifying activities, dignified care seemed to emerge. By "modifying," I'm referring to when a physical therapist or a wheelchair vendor would manipulate a material object to improve fit. During Dean's AT Clinic session, approximately 20 minutes into the appointment, the first instance of a measure+modify practice

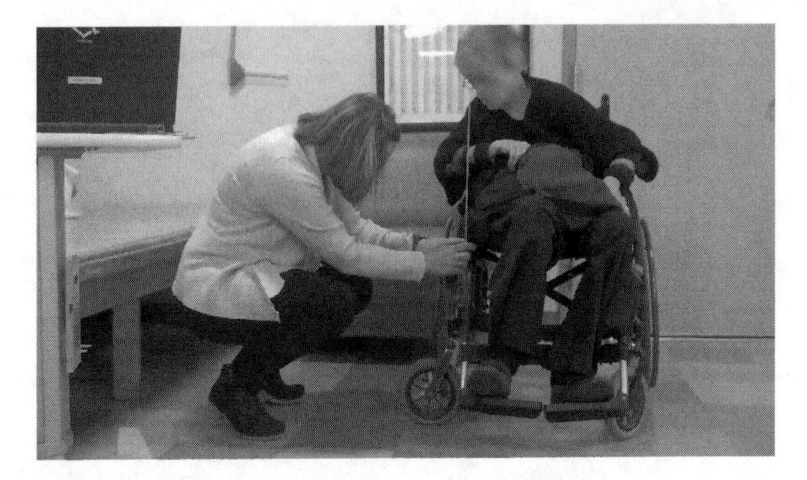

Figure 4.6. Stephanie uses a yardstick to take a measurement from Hazel's new wheelchair.

took place. Scott measured sitting pressure with a sensor-filled seat mat connected by a cord to his laptop. After placing the mat under Dean's buttocks, Scott could see on his computer screen those areas where Dean's contact with the seat portended the possibility of pressure sores. After a few (self-deprecating) jokes from Loretta about how glad she was that *her* bottom wasn't being visualized, Scott went on to pair measurement with modification.

Based on the measurements he saw on the screen, Scott repositioned the seat cushion, the pressure-mapping mat, and the wheelchair (by elevating the seat, tilting the back, etc.) to find a good fit for Dean. The three panels of figures 4.7 are still images from this iterative process of measuring and modifying while using pressure-mapping software to guide shifts of position to relieve pressure.

The excerpt below exemplifies the measure+modify practice (note the presence of show+teach as well). Pay special attention to the silences.

SCOTT: So, this is a picture of your bottom on the cushion. Okay? I'm taking pictures of your bottom. [Scott places both hands on his buttocks]

[Dean, Loretta, and Scott laugh]

SCOTT: Okay. So, this is like a weather map. You have, you know, whites and blues and yellows and reds; you want to kind of avoid the reds and oranges and yellows if you can because that indicates higher pressure . . . and there's a 3D map over here that you can look at too. There's this one spot here. And I got a feeling that might not be your bones. It might actually be the mat kind of twisted underneath you a little bit . . . This just gives you an idea of where the pressure mostly is in your bottom. Your left leg is here, your right leg is here. Your right bottom cheek is there, your left bottom cheek is there. So, there's that area of high pressure, and there's more pressure at the back, which makes sense if that's where you're carrying most of your weight. So, if you can just hang on, I'm going to try and straighten this mat out underneath you. Can you lean forward for a moment? Ok. And then back down. That's great.

[Crinkly sound of protective plastic cover rubbing on mat]

SCOTT: There we go. Yeah. It's probably more normal. I would say. I'm gonna take a picture of that.

[Seven seconds of silence while Scott types on his laptop]

SCOTT: [places his right hand on laptop mouse, bends at waist while standing to face the laptop screen] How's that feel?

DEAN: Ok.

[Twelve seconds of silence while Scott types on his laptop]

DEAN: How long will it take me to mentally and physically adapt to this? You know what I'm trying to say? Like, a learning curve?

SCOTT: [stands up, turns toward Dean and away from laptop screen] Yeah, well, the first day is just training. [reaches nondominant left hand out to lean on his mobile laptop desk, places his other hand on his hip, and crosses one ankle over the other in a casual stance]. And you'll get really good at it when you use it a lot, you know, but for right now it's my job to sort of just make it . . .

DEAN: [interrupts] I've seen people full speed, you know? But they did it for a while.

SCOTT: Yeah. [smiles] Yeah.

[Dean smiles back]

SCOTT: Yes, you'll get used to it. I think my job is to help you get comfortable with it, with the basics, right?

[Dean nods repeatedly]

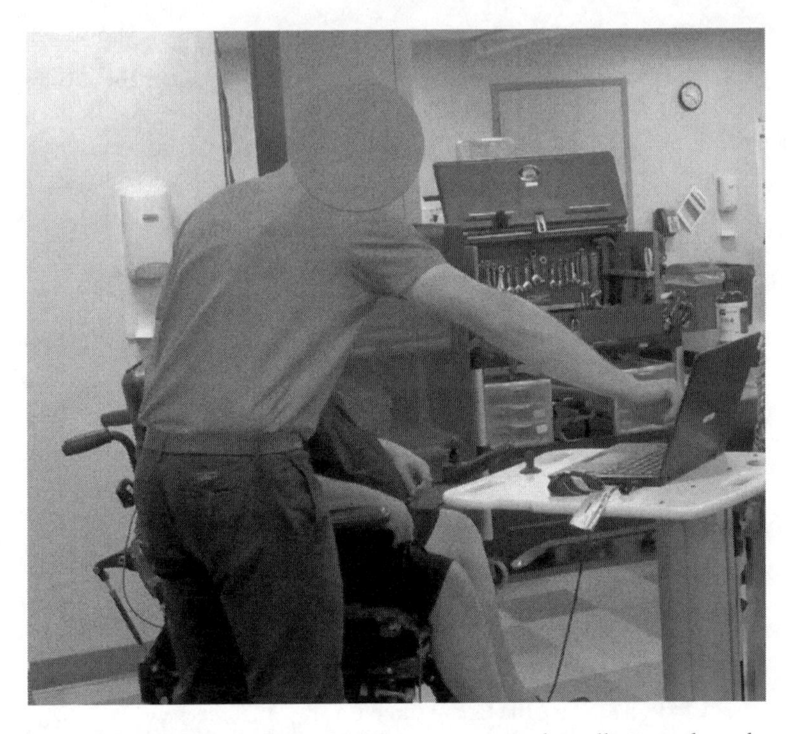

Figures 4.7. Scott puts measure+modify into practice as he walks Dean through pressure mapping with the goal of increasing Dean's comfort (*here* and *opposite*).

SCOTT: And then make sure that you're safe within environments that you're used to—like home environments, communities.

[Dean nods again]

SCOTT: But we can do training too, so if you feel like you're not comfortable driving the chair at first, you can come back and see me and we can just practice. [gestures with right hand in loop shape that connects him at his waist with Dean's upper body]

[Dean nods again]

SCOTT: But [grins] we don't know how good you'll do if you haven't even started.

[Dean grins and looks down; Scott turns to face his laptop screen]

I include this excerpt not just because it illustrates the practice of measure+modify in pressure mapping but also because it includes one of the

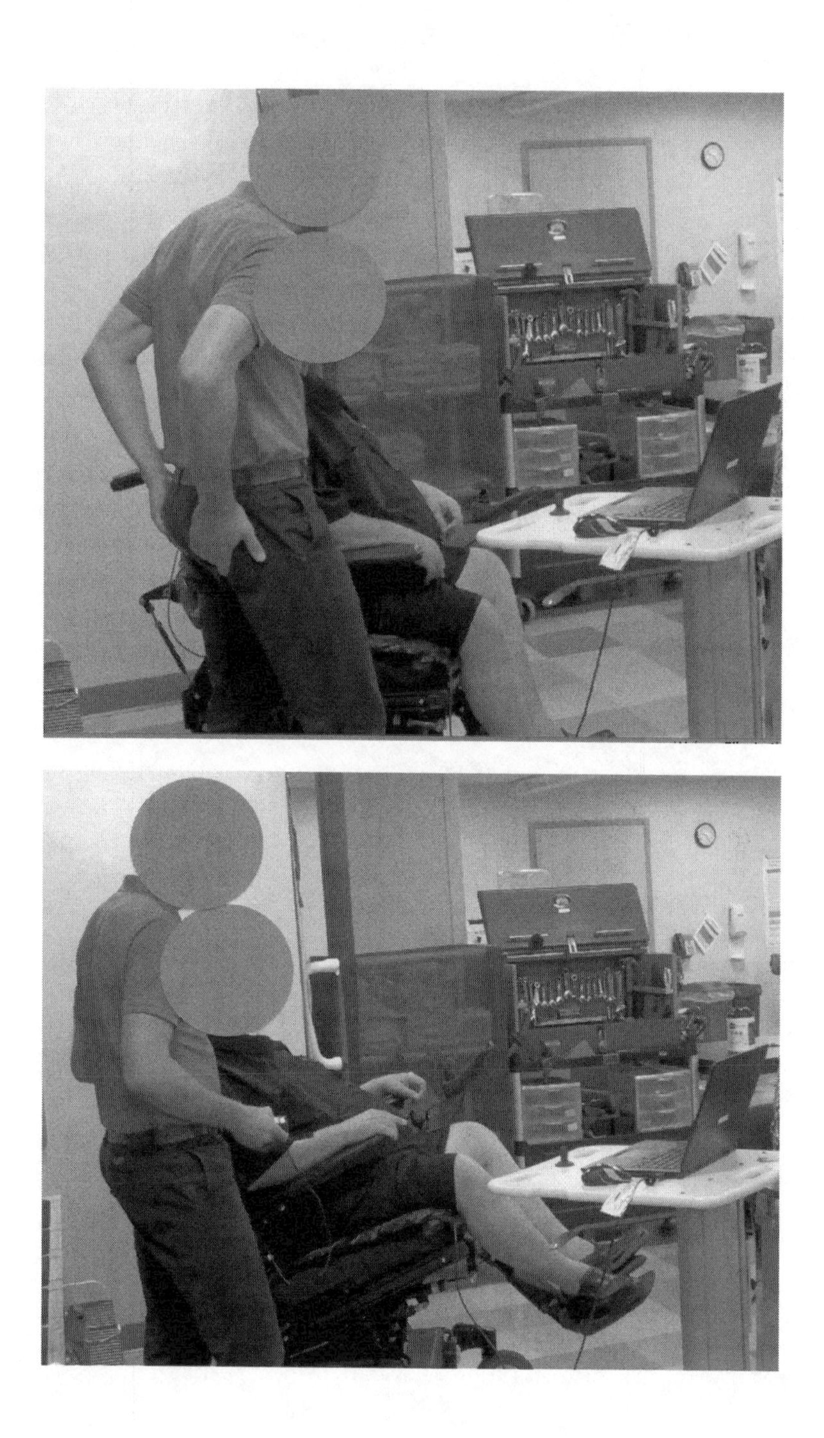

longest periods of silence I observed across all AT Clinic sessions. The silence opens space for Dean hesitantly to wonder aloud about how long it will take him to get used to a new chair. The 12 seconds of silence I mark in the excerpt are meaningful since, as Ellingson (2017) notes, "silences are . . . not merely the absence of speech but embodied practices" (p. 95). If, following Ellingson's guidance, I "attend not only to the overt activity . . . but to the spaces in between that help to give those activities meaning," I'm able to inquire about the nature of this silence (p. 95). This silence ushered in the only time during the appointment when Dean explicitly expressed an affective concern without his daughter, Loretta, interceding in some way.

Scott's willingness to tinker with the pressure-mapping tool, while pointing out to Dean where parts of his body were represented on the screen, provided enough quiet, empty space for Dean to wonder out loud about potential contingencies; moreover, Scott's patient tinkering conveyed his desire to make multiple adjustments to fit in response to Dean's positionality. In these micro-moments, the AT Clinic becomes what rhetoricians might characterize as "a 'dwelling place' (*ethos*) where people can take the time to deliberate and 'know-together' (*conscientia*) some topic of interest and, in the process, perhaps gain a more authentic understanding of, and feel more at home with, those who are willing to contribute to its development" (Hyde & McSpiritt, 2007, p. 159). Perhaps not quite "access intimacy" (Mingus, 2011), dwelling carves out rhetorical space for finding fit. Finding the right fit requires an ongoing and iterative willingness to acknowledge an Other's exposedness: "Acknowledgment requires a sustained openness to others even if, at times, things become boring or troublesome" (Hyde, 2006, pp. 3–4). When compared to the rest of Dean's session, this moment stands out for how Dean has space to imagine himself in a new wheelchair and to consider potential challenges associated with transitioning to it. By making explicit his commitment to remain responsive to new arrangements (however temporary or fleeting), Scott creates the conditions whereby dignified care can emerge. "Adaptations," as Mol (2021) notes, "form the hallmark of caring kinds of *doing*" (p. 87). As I'll describe in the next chapter, contrary to the feel-goodness of the rhetorical "dwelling place" (Hyde & Mc-

Spiritt), though, doing dignity anticipates, recognizes, and responds to when a fit feels "off." This, too, requires adaptation.

The above analysis of the four paired practices demonstrated how finding a good-enough-for-now fit highlights the "obligation, imperative, or moment of addressivity—the real time recognition of one another's exposure to exposedness" (Davis, 2010, p. 11). Indeed, "having to be in communication means being exposed," which may cause one to wonder, "How will my words and actions be perceived? Do I make sense? Will I be recognized?" (Butchart 2019, p. 13). It's in these anxious worries about one's rhetoricity that conditions for un/dignified care arise. The practice of responding to a wheelchair user's desires "is not a matter of deeds ostensibly done well" but rather is a negotiation of a good-enough-for-now fit, which "requires recursive attentiveness to what happens as an unintentional consequence of one's *doings*" (Mol, 2021, p. 99).

In the AT Clinic, conditions for dignified care emerged when it was clear to Stephanie and Scott that *not* responding "is *not* an option" (Davis, 2010, p. 12; emphasis mine). They attempted to find a good-enough-for-now fit by responding to a host of corporeal contingencies through (at least) four practices. Hazel's exposedness was evident in her own internalized ableism. Dean's exposedness was apparent in his desire to maintain independence in a world that sees his body's size and disability as presenting an uninsurable "wildcard" that requires paying out of pocket. In another patient's case, whose story was not included in this chapter, their exposedness was evidenced by an impending divorce that threatened to radically change his wheelchair options upon a downgrading of insurance coverage. AT Clinic patients' embodied exposedness was on full display. Over and over again, physical therapists, mobility industry vendors, and even family members had "to *do* one's very best, acknowledge failure, take a step back, and begin again" (Mol, 2021, p. 100). Some of these care practices may, at first glance, seem small or insignificant. Yet their accumulation over time results in a kind of practical repertoire of dignified care. Taken together, such practices honor a person's exposedness despite the ways that market-driven medicine attempts to force a good-enough-for-now-fit as a long-term solution.

CHAPTER FIVE

Dignified Care as Ethical Praxis

> Start, stop, begin again, but in a different way.
>
> —*Annemarie Mol,* Eating in Theory

I struggled with a lot of things while drafting this book. One of the biggest was verb tense. For example, I remained unsure about what tense to use in my discussion of COVID-19. Do I speak about the COVID-19 pandemic as past? Will it be over by the time this book goes to press? I took care not refer to the COVID-19 pandemic as *the* pandemic since such shorthand might cause future readers to ask, "Which one?" By the time *Doing Dignity* is published, there might well be another pandemic upon us. As I write this, COVID-19 indeed persists, and my immunocompromised partner and I remain relatively isolated while many of our friends and families carry on with "business as usual" (Scuro, 2017, p. 113). Like the study participants described in chapter two, we remain prone—disoriented by competing forces that, by forcefully and unendingly acting on us, keep us in flux.

To address such disorienting existential pronation, in chapter two I offered two constructs that index COVID-19's necropolitical mangle: un/dignified asides and bedside in/dignities. Un/dignified asides are the "contextual matters" that are "often omitted from medical ethics discussions that focus on individual cases, largely because they fade into the background and are simply assumed rather than examined" (Groenhout,

2019, p. 23). Examining the particularities of such contextual matters allowed me to account for the perpetual pronation and existential disorientation of health care providers (HCPs) during a global health crisis where "systems of inequality" were (and are . . . *see what I mean?!*) more evident than ever (Gupta, 2020, p. 2). Composite narratives from Edna, Kai, Luca, Idris, and Naomi provided insight into how a host of infrastructural inheritances and preexisting conditions intra-acted (Barad, 2003, 2007) with local logics of care/lessness in ways that (continue to) shape COVID-19 caretaking. Doing dignity in such situations seemed impossible most of the time given the constraints with which care frequently collided. HCPs appeared caught in a double bind of having to contend with undignified infrastructural inheritances even as they themselves were complicit in such structures.[1] As a result, a kind of existential weariness emerged.

Chapter three transitioned from the HCP experience with COVID-19 caretaking to state-level politics of care/lessness by examining recent Medical Aid in Dying (MAiD) legislative hearings in Nevada and Connecticut. By tracing the biopolitical topoi that underwrote testimony, I uncovered how some ordinary people (perhaps unwittingly) pathologized dependency when justifying their stance on MAiD. If we consider how such local (bedside) logics of care/lessness might be scaled up into actual policy—what Scuro (2017) calls "ideologies with political teeth" (p. xxx)—we see more clearly how local in/dignities accrete over time to yield state-level necropolitics that, once operationalized, churn out another vicious cycle of intra-acting un/dignified asides and in/dignities at the bedside. What results is the state-sanctioned "authorized disposability" of certain persons, including those who are elderly, disabled, unhoused, or without kinship networks (Jackson, 2016, p. 19). Doing dignity requires confronting, calling out, or at the very least recognizing, as Mr. Gillums from chapter three did, local logics of care/lessness that are animated, at best, by a feigned universality or, at worst, by an "indifference to difference" (Mbembe, 2019, p. 59).

Chapter four focused on care-in-practice at a hospital's assistive technology clinic (AT Clinic). Through close analysis of how care was (em)bodied by "small, ineffable gestures" (Diedrich, 2019, p. 589), I identified four key practices that seeded conditions conducive to in/dignity during

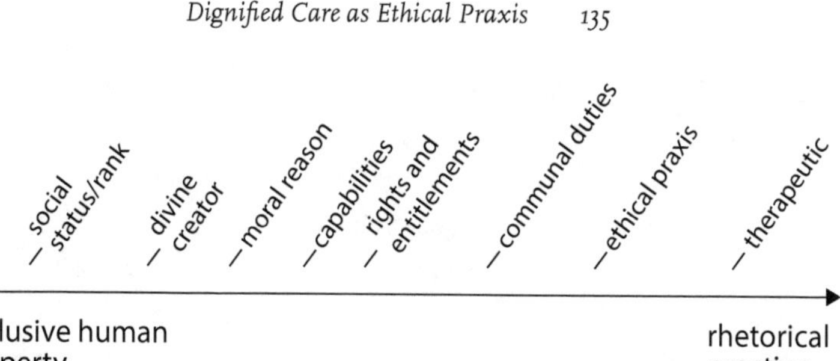

Figure 5.1. A continuum of dignity's mechanisms, ranging from dignity posited as an exclusive human property (*left*) to dignity posited as a rhetorical practice (*right*).

Hazel's and Dean's wheelchair fitting appointments. Physical therapists enacted rhetorical and clinical skills in response to trans-corporeal (Alaimo, 2008) contingencies that emerged during otherwise quotidian care-in-practice micro-moments. Ultimately, chapter four illustrated how un/dignified care is an iterative practice that involves finding a good-enough-for-now fit by recognizing and responding to another's "exposedness" (Davis, 2010, p. 11).

Taken together, results from the chapters' analyses of un/dignified care inform a practice account of dignity that eschews premodern and Enlightenment notions of human dignity—notions that, as chapter one described them, hinge on hierarchical humanhoods. Recall chapter one's discussion of dignity's harmful biopolitical ancestry in relation to figure 5.1, which illustrates (rudimentarily) how dignity might be theorized as existing on a continuum, where one end is dignity-as-a-property-of-humanhood and the other end is dignity-as-a-rhetorical-practice. Ranging between these two poles are different sources of dignity plotted along the connecting axis. This continuum unfortunately suggests linearity, but nothing about dignity's emergence as witnessed in my case studies was linear.

At the left end of the continuum, dignity derives from an exclusive, intrinsic property of human being. At the right end of the continuum, dignity derives from rhetorical practice. I situate Greco-Roman dignity, which was conferred through mechanisms of social status or rank, far to the left. As discussed in chapter one, theories of dignity were later thought to be divinely bestowed by a benevolent God. Kantian notions of dignity then emerged as the coin of the realm, with a person's moral capacity for reason being the primary mechanism by which dignity was warranted. Neo-Kantian notions of dignity have since taken hold, as exemplified by, for example, Martha Nussbaum's (2008) capabilities approach. Multivocal notions of dignity in our contemporary moment form the basis through which human rights and state-guaranteed entitlements are legitimated. I plot non-Western communitarian approaches to dignity on the right side of the continuum because they move us toward a dignity that is more of a communal act to which duties of care are attendant. Finally, I hypothesize that dignity as ethical praxis is an unabashedly rhetorical practice—far removed from an exclusive, individual, or inherent property of human being.

The qualities and characteristics of doing dignity as a rhetorical practice are most akin to Nora Jacobson's (2012) theory of "social dignity." A complement to "human dignity," "social dignity" is "characterized by the push and pull between fixity and flexibility, between ideal and actual, between relation to self and relation to others" (p. 18). It is "generated in action and interaction" (p. 17) and distinct from the other types of dignity Jacobson describes in the introduction to her book *Dignity and Health.*[2] Motivated by Allen's (2018) definition of rhetorical theory as "the self-consciously ethical study of how symbolic animals negotiate constraint," I extend Jacobson's "social dignity" a step further to focus on how social dignity is practiced when negotiating constraint. Importantly, though, Jacobson identifies social dignity as both "scalable and contingent: it can be measured and compared, violated and promoted" (p. 17). Building from Jacobson's claim that dignity can be promoted, I conclude this chapter with the possibility of doing dignity as a therapeutic practice, which I situate on the far right of the spectrum.

But first, let's review three general propositions I center in a practice account of dignity:

1. *Doing* dignity highlights how care-in-practice (Mol, Moser, & Pols, 2015) is continually caught between the particularities of local logics of care/lessness and larger biopolitical inheritances—specifically, what I call "un/dignified asides" and "in/dignities at the bedside."

2. *Doing* dignity requires us to "demystify the universalist pretentions of Western humanism" (Mbembe, 2019, p. 161) by recognizing and redressing humanhood's harmful biopolitical ancestry.
3. *Doing* dignity never absolves us of the ways our approaches to care-in-practice are complicit in local and structural care/lessness. Anything but heroic, doing dignity requires an ethical disposition toward "thought-reflection-action, and thought-reflection on this action." (Walsh & Mignolo, 2018, p. 7)

Thus far, I have described how each case study illustrates proposition 1. In what follows, I provide more backing for proposition 2 and unpack in detail proposition 3.

Proposition 2. *Doing dignity requires us to "demystify the universalist pretentions of Western humanism" by recognizing and redressing humanhood's harmful biopolitical ancestry.* Some of contemporary caretaking's most idealized principles and platitudes have roots in hierarchical humanhoods that discriminate, devalue, and debilitate, even as they cl/aim to uplift, value, and empower (see Antonovich, 2021; Lynch, 2019). I began this book by criticizing how, in an otherwise good-willed attempt at building coalition, we selectively respond to spectacular displays of suffering that circulate virally via logics of hierarchical humanhood. Embedded in critiques of sentimentalized solidarity is cynicism about what critical Black studies calls "universal humanity" (Jackson, 2020, p. 29)—a category of hierarchical humanhood that works by situating "certain people (white, male, able-bodied) within greater or lesser proximity to humanness" (King, 2017, p. 165). Critical feminist posthumanists have leveraged a similar critique of "the human." Here is Braidotti's (2020) summary of the matter:

> Not all humans are equal and the human is not at all a neutral category. It is rather a normative category that indexes access to privileges and entitlements. Appeals to the "human" are always discriminatory: they create structural distinctions and inequalities among different categories of humans. Humanity is a quality that is distributed according to a hierarchical scale centered on a humanistic idea of Man as the measure of all things. This dominant idea is based on a simple assumption of superiority by a subject that is: masculine, white, Eurocentric, practicing compulsory het-

> erosexuality and reproduction, able-bodied, urbanized, speaking a standard language. This subject is the Man of reason that feminists, anti-racists, black, indigenous postcolonial and ecological activists have been criticizing for decades. (p. 466)

Modern-day displays and fetishizations of unity are attempts at absolving the human (read: me) from our (read: my) harmful biopolitical ancestry. Rhetorical moves to universalize human suffering insidiously provide a pass for the routine logics of classification that result in some persons' biopolitical disposability, as we saw in the MAiD deliberations described in chapter three. These logics of classification scale up to policies that replicate harmful "misrecognition(s) of human kinship" (Wynter, 1994, p. 15).

How such logics of misrecognition scale up over time into a necropolitical apparatus that governs some persons' slow death (Berlant, 2007) or social death (Hyde, 2006) is a point Wynter (1994) drives home with a profound example: the Los Angeles Police Department's use of the acronym NHI, standing for "No Humans Involved," in official police reporting of the beating of Rodney King. Criminal indifference does not always manifest as obviously as discursive markers like NHI. A more insidious genre of criminal indifference might look like Derek Chauvin's courtroom defense, which relied on "expert" physician testimony attributing George Floyd's death to heart disease and fentanyl use, not to the knee pressing down on his neck for nine minutes. Such expert testimony is palimpsestic of the early 1900s when Black men who were accused of rape were medically castrated since, "physicians argued, white America would come to prefer the tidiness of medical punishments over the unruliness of mob lynchings" (Antonovich, 2021, p. 439). Indeed, modern medicine has a long legacy of "ritual violence" (Murray, 2022, p. 26), including modern allopathic gynecology's foundation on brutal experiments conducted on enslaved Black women who were thought to feel less pain than white women (Dudley, 2012). Modern medicine's legacy of "ritual violence" also includes the human genome project's scientific racism.[3]

A practice account of dignity must address the multiscalar violence caused by "Man's" logics of misrecognition. But it should do more than just offer an indictment. It must provide pathways for a different version of dignity, ones pointing toward the "new genre of being human" endorsed by Sylvia Wynter (2003, p. 269). I therefore imagine dignified care as a form of ethical praxis—an ethical disposition that "envisions the human as a verb, as alterable, as relational" (McKittrick, 2015, p. 7). The possibility for such pathways ought not to be misinterpreted as some type of idealized "born again" moment, mind you (cf. Colebrook, 2020, p. 380). Instead, what I humbly suggest is a kind of asymptotic posture (Allen, 2018) of ethical praxis that iteratively reflects on, responds to, and renegotiates constraint. We must "start, stop, begin again, but in a different way" (Mol, 2021, p. 142). Importantly, dignified care as ethical praxis ought not to be construed as the "Capitalocene," which "allow(s) humanity to be a virtuous and virtual remainder that might rise, like a phoenix from the ashes, having broken from its grubby past" (Colebrook, p. 380). Backing for such an anticipatory rebuttal will unfold next as I unpack proposition 3 by offering a personal story that illustrates contemporary caretaking's harmful entanglements and rhetoricity's "two-wayness."

Proposition 3. *Doing dignity never absolves us of the ways our approaches to care-in-practice are complicit in local and structural care/lessness. Anything but heroic, doing dignity requires an ethical disposition toward "thought-reflection-action, and thought-reflection on this action."* Each case study in this book dove deeply into some of the material-discursive conditions (i.e., in/dignities at and beyond the bedside) that conspire with and permit an "indifference to difference" (Mbembe, 2019, p. 59). Each chapter illustrated how rhetoricity is entangled with "relational senses of self and responsibility"; accordingly, human being "centres on a concern with ethical praxis and the practical connectivities which secure the well-being of those least mobile and most vulnerable, *not* as discursive subject positions, but as mortal others-in-relation" (Whatmore, 1997, p. 44). A practice account of dignity, then, requires an ethical obligation to mortal others-in-relation. Such an ethical obligation must be neither indifferent to nor sentimental about difference. Allow me to share a two-part personal story that I hope illustrates what this ethical obligation to mortal others-in-relation might look like.

Part 1. Back in 2018, my partner had a serious surgical operation, which resulted in a weeklong hospital stay at the Cleveland Clinic. One night, as I waited in my partner's room for his return from undergoing one of many tests, a man in his mid-fifties was rolled into the room on a gurney. For the next few hours, multiple HCPs came and went, setting him up in his new bed. I wasn't trying to eavesdrop, but I couldn't help but hear the goings-on a few feet away behind a partitioning curtain. I overheard that this man had spent the last week in the intensive care unit. He'd had a stroke and was now unable to walk, use the bathroom, or be heard well enough for people to know he was saying "Bill"—not "Mill"—when they asked for his name.

Over the next five days, every single time a new HCP or environmental or dining services staffer entered the room and said to (not asked) Bill, "How are you," he answered them, much to the person's surprise. And his answer was the same every time: a jovial, if not exuberant, "*I'm alive!*" Immediately following Bill's "*I'm alive!*" was an awkward pause. Occasionally, there'd be a chuckle. It seemed like no one quite knew how to respond to Bill's answer. But the pressure *to* respond was palpable. After about the tenth time I witnessed Bill's ritual response, I started to consider the possibility that his assertion was more than just dry-witted literalism. Instead, I imagined that Bill's "*I'm alive*" may as well have ended with ". . . *dammit!*" Every person who entered H-151, room 12 was put on notice: Bill is, indeed, alive. Acknowledge him, dammit.

One way to understand Bill's declaration is as a demand for "affirmation and validation," what rhetoricians describe as "communicative behavior that grants attention to others and thereby makes room for them in our lives" (Hyde, 2006, pp. xvi, 1). These openings, responses, forms of recognition, and acknowledgment—these are the spaces where rhetoricity emerges. Rhetoricity, then, requires heightened attunement to our entanglements, or "dwelling spaces" that "found our communal relationships with others" (Hyde, p. 56), even (perhaps especially) during routine bedside rituals. Following Levinas, Katie Oliviero (2018) describes a "pre-originary *susceptiveness* [to the other] which chooses me before I welcome it," but importantly, this susceptiveness is "dialogical," which indexes the "two-wayness of reciprocity" (p. 133).

To fully unpack rhetoricity's two-wayness, allow me to highlight what I see as a meaningful distinction between recognition and acknowledgment: "People often speak of these two phenomena as if they were one in the same . . . *Recognition is only a preliminary step* in this process of attuning one's consciousness toward another" (Hyde, 2006, p. 3; emphasis added). More capacious than recognition, acknowledgment, Hyde suggests, is what "provides openings and thus more living room for people in the thickets of existence"—what he calls a kind of "ethical . . . home-making" (pp. 19, 117). Akin to Hyde's home-making is Davis's (2005) "radically hospitable opening to alterity" (p. 207). These forms of radical hospitality confer rhetorical acknowledgment, while recognition is more provisional, a cautious first step. It may seem like I'm splitting hairs by distinguishing between mere rhetorical *recognition* and a more radical *acknowledgment*. To understand why I'm making this distinction, let's return to Bill's bedside.

Part 2. On about my third day at the Cleveland Clinic, around the time I noticed that no family or friends had come to visit Bill, and after I had witnessed numerous conversational "lurches and spasms" (Davis, 2017, p. 434) in response to Bill's attempts at (demi)rhetoricity, I overheard him making sexual advances to the nurse tasked with bathing him. Mortified, the nurse abruptly ended Bill's bath and fled the room. My concern shifted away from Bill and toward his nurse. I wondered whether she had a history of sexual or gender-based violence and whether this experience might have triggered her. I wondered if she had someone she could talk to about what happened once she got home. I wondered if she would report the incident. I wondered if maybe I should report the incident.

For the rest of the week, whenever my partner was wheeled away for another test, I walked the hallways instead of staying in the room with Bill. The "fragility" of rhetoricity's "horizonless and ungatherable 'world'" that is "opened each time in the address of the other" was horrifyingly palpable that week (Davis, 2017, p. 434). What I witnessed while sharing a room with Bill was the perpetual collision of varying vulnerability. I felt like I had a front-row seat to a host of human sufferings as they unfolded in real time.

Here's the thing, though: Initially, when I recounted this story about Bill on paper, I wrote only the first part. Bill's disability, corporeal fragility, and aloneness shaped how I (sentimentally) (re)constructed his demi-rhetoricity. I'm guessing I also may have been projecting my partner's own health struggles onto Bill's. Maybe I'm even feeling embarrassed or ashamed about how easily my empathy for Bill was replaced by concern for his nurse, as if caring is a zero-sum game that can only be justified by absolute innocence. I wasn't reminded of the other half of the Bill story until after I had transcribed the interview with Kai from chapter two where he shared an experience of caring for a patient who said racist things:

> And you're just like holy, like . . . All right, I didn't know we were going down that road. I really don't want to talk about that with you. I have extremely different views on this than you. But even though all of that is true, it doesn't change the underlying fact, which is I'm here to be a provider for you, and you have real needs. And because of that I should do everything within my power to prevent anything from disrupting that care because that's, that's my mission.

One of the goals of this project—the project of *doing dignity,* that is—is to tell the *other* half of the story about Bill. Not all "dwelling spaces" ripe for acknowledgment are safe. Both Kai's caretaking experience and the story about Bill (the *full* story) illustrate rhetoricity's risks and the stakes of care. Yes, there are power dynamics at work in contemporary caretaking. Indeed, health care professionals "have the social permission and responsibility to determine what forms of existence are 'abnormal' and how various 'abnormalities' are to be managed" (Ho, 2011, p. 108). But to assume that Bill's nurse or Kai must endure such harm simply because they are in a position of power simply doubles down on the rank-based hierarchies critiqued in chapter one.

So, what am I suggesting here? That there are more (or less) ethical ways of responding to certain forms of material-discursive violence? That care requires some necessary harms to which we must acquiesce? Neither actually. By telling both parts of the story, I am attempting to resist the spectacular and sentimental rhetorics that emerge from our entangled, interdependent condition. The temptation to romanticize our entanglements, in other words, can also perpetuate harm. Each of this book's case studies has demonstrated how contemporary caretaking is fraught with a host of in/dignities at and beyond the bedside. Telling both parts of the Bill story highlights the "two-wayness of reciprocity" (Oliviero, 2018, p. 133). The option exists, even for Hyde, of not responding. My aim here is to affirm that some entanglements do indeed result in (mutual) harm.

In fact, harm need not always manifest itself in interpersonal abuse. HCPs' continual exposure to exposedness, as documented in chapter two, resulted in a kind of inner existential harm, or what participant after participant described as burnout:

> I think if somebody in my work was lacking the ability to provide dignified care during COVID, it would come out in the form of burnout. So, it wouldn't be an intentional, you know, it wouldn't be intentional; it would be them, or anybody on the team, not checking in with themselves and not realizing they're burnt out . . . I feel often that they need more then we're able to give. And we don't have the volunteers anymore and you don't have the family members, and it's just, you know, you try to be more than adequate but sometimes it's . . . I would leave work and just be kind of shaking and tired walking across the parking lot and think, "I'm not wearing an N95 mask. I'm not taking care of COVID-positive patients, and I feel just overwhelmed." (Focus Group Participant, 12/17/2020)

HCPs' burnout is a form of Levinasian "weariness" that emerges when "existence is like the reminder of a commitment to exist, with all the seriousness and harshness of an unrevokable contract . . . Weariness is the impossible refusal of this ultimate obligation" (Levinas, qtd. in Hyde, 2006, p. 121). It's a kind of "suffocating embrace" that "incites fatigue" (p. 121). Specifically, "in order to hold off the abject weariness of existence, we must do things that are prone to make us tired and weary over time. It is the 'myth of Sisyphus,' *for real*" (p. 121). Weariness emerges as a result of "being directly exposed to being" (Levinas, qtd. on p. 120). Such weariness causes suffering, which Levinas says, "is made up of the impossibility of fleeing or retreating. The whole acuity of suffering lies in this impossibility of retreat. It is the fact of being backed up against life and being" (qtd. on p. 120). As ballast to burnout, doing dignity provides a flexible "disposition" (Lundberg & Gunn, 2005, p. 98)—an ethical praxis that is sensitized to the risky business of being exposed to exposedness.

Such a disposition is rhetorical. It involves what Heard (2013) describes as an "attunement" that "postures us to respond to the other even as we recognize the incompleteness of our response" (p. 61). The incompleteness of our response is the point, actually. Alluding to the in-progress nature of a nonhierarchical humanhood, Wynter describes the human as "less a name than a praxis and a becoming" (qtd. In Mbembe, 2019, p. 160).[4] Praxis as "a becoming" affirms the fact of fit's good-enough-for-now nature and remains "open to the possibility of being shocked, surprised, and overwhelmed" as we repeatedly engage "with alterity" (Heard, pp. 45, 46). The thing toward which we are always becoming is a "new genre of the human" (Wynter, 1994) that flourishes within "novel assemblages of relation" (Weheliye, 2014, p. 13). Such novel assemblages of relation might be, I humbly hope, mediated by ethical praxis, wherein praxis is "thought-reflection-action, and thought-reflection on this action" (Walsh & Mignolo, 2018, p. 7). In other words, praxis is not just the yoking of theory with practice. It is a disposition that involves iterative reflection, rethinking, and re-acting, or as Mol (2021) writes, "negotiating, tinkering, trying, and trying again" (p. 77).

Recall from chapter one Allen's (2018) definition of rhetoric as "the self-consciously ethical study of how symbolic animals negotiate constraint" (p. 4). Emboldening rhetoric's self-consciousness is what I see as Walsh and Mignolo's (2018) "thought-reflection-action, and thought-reflection on this action" (p. 7). And what we're working toward in all our self-conscious, Wynterian "becoming" involves a few intermediary steps: specifically, being "less awful at *living together in a world structured by divisions*" (Allen, p. 273; emphasis in the original). What I am suggesting by locating parallels between Wynter's new genre of the human, Allen's ethical fantasy, and Walsh and Mignolo's praxis is a version of dignified care that might be described as "troubled freedom" (Allen, p. 269). Re-seeing dignified care as troubled freedom paves the way for an emancipatory Wynterian future, but it is not that future. Allen employs the analogy of the "asymptote" to describe how "we do not reach troubled freedom but only approach it, seeking not certainty, metaphysical or otherwise, but truthfully less dissatisfying inhibitions of satisfaction"; he goes on to say, "Rhetorical theory aims for workability, with an over-the-long-haul horizon entailing an ever-enlarged community of freedom" (Allen, p. 272). Dignified care, then, is an asymptotic, temporarily workable solution—

always only good-enough-for-now—and hinges on right response to a host of trans-corporeal constraints (Alaimo 2008, 2018).

By "right response" I am invoking Louise Wetherbee Phelps (1991), who, in her discussion of *phronesis*, characterizes "right action" as dependent on a situation's particularities (p. 864). I'm also reminded of my frustration with the Al-Anon slogan "Do the next right thing," to which I at one time exasperatedly responded, "Yeah, but *how do I know* what's right?!" Now, I realize I'm always a step behind in being persuaded of what the next right thing is, will, or could even be. "Persuasion, then, is a matter of our 'acknowledging' the pattern of accumulated particulars" (Hyde, 2006, p. 80). That is, by reflecting on the consequences and effects of previous attempts at doing the next right thing, we are tenuously persuaded to seed future right responses. As Boyle (2018) asserts, "practice makes persuasion" (p. 55).

There are, in fact, times when right response invites certain forms of quotidian bedside duties. But there will be other times when right response will need to involve radical responsivity, even resistance. "Right" response, then, isn't yet another sentimental or idealized human reaction. Right response, depending on the particularities of the situation, may in fact call for not-responding. Not-responding is a form of non-indifference (which is different from a non-response predicated on indifference to difference). Consider Scuro's (2017) example of not-responding: "there needs to be . . . a kind of *caretaker prescience*—an insight and foresight for when to assist and advocate, and when to 'stand down' (or, even STFU [shut the f*ck up])" (p. 16). This description of non-response is one alternative to what Scuro describes as "receptive affection," which involves "an openness to the other . . . to not be averse to the foreign and nonnormative . . . an approach more like an 'awakening' and 'vigilance' " (p. 18). Non-response might also take the form of silence. Silence, or what Karenga (2013) says might better be termed "restraint," was indeed one of premodern Egypt's five rhetorical canons (n.p.).[5] The point here is that not all responses require the kind of radical acknowledgment Hyde calls for. In fact, doing dignity may also look at times like "doing nothing" or "letting go" (Mol, 2021, p. 88).

Lack of discernment about whom we give acknowledgment can also result in a slow or social death. For example, in our attempts at undoing the exclusionary, calculative approach to "universal humanity" critiqued in chapter one, (white) sentimentality may result in the impulse to hurtle ahead at full speed into romanticized ethics of entanglement. Without resisting that impulse, we may swing so far in the opposite direction that we enact a different kind of indifference to difference—a brand of human dignity that fails to "function in relation with limits" (Allen, 2005, p. 6). Even Barad's (2007) notion of entanglement requires the "enactment of boundaries and exclusions" to ensure "the ongoing reconfiguring of the space of possibilities for future enactments" (p. 391). Aware of rhetoricity's risk, Giraud (2019) goes as far as to advocate for an ethics of exclusion. For Giraud, an ethics of exclusion might act as ballast against the instability wrought when relations are damaging and when care sometimes "shore[s] up inequalities" (p. 117). Giraud is careful to clarify that exclusion does not necessarily signify a "negation"; rather, exclusions, limits, boundaries—they enable a constitutive and creative reimagining of contemporary caretaking: "although nothing might exist outside of relation, *certain* things might need distance from *certain* relations" (pp. 171–173). Rhetorically, the kind of ethics of exclusion Giraud advocates can be actualized by withholding radical acknowledgment, choosing to "stand down" or even to "STFU" (Scuro, 2017, p. 16).

Thus far I have argued that dignified care as ethical praxis—which, as a reminder, requires a rhetorical disposition toward "thought-reflection-action, and thought-reflection on this action" (Walsh & Mignolo, 2018, p. 7)—may over time reveal patterns of harm owing to our "primordial state of proximity" (Hyde, 2006, p. 132). By providing more detail about contemporary caretaking's harmful entanglements and rhetoricity's two-wayness, I hope to have justified why we need a theory of dignified care that still finds value in self-reflection and even in the idea of a "self" at all. Indeed, the self, or "the *I* that *is*," is what "exchanges materials with [one's] surroundings through semipermeable boundaries" (Mol, 2021, p. 142). Needed now, as we work toward "better ways of attuning to other creatures and the earth" (Mol, p. 137), is an ethical praxis that re-values rhetorical practices associated with iterative reflection, rethinking, and re-acting. We need the "I" for an ethics capable of accounting for the fact that "I may want to do the right thing . . . but, one way or another, what

I do may turn out to be bad" (p. 101). Such an ethic does not offer "reassuring handholds," nor does it "envision this or that goal in isolation"; instead, it "realizes that deeds inevitably have diverse effects" (p. 101). Disrupting "dreams of global equivalence" need "not mean that *thinking* . . . deserves scorn" (pp. 138, 140; emphasis added).

Allow me to parse the difference between a "self" and the liberal humanist notion of "the individual." Neoliberal individualism is simply the other side of the "universal humanity" coin. The very idea of *doing* dignity should not be misconstrued as a romanticized, neoliberal replacement for eroding (if not eradicated) systems of social support. As the Care Collective (2020) has noted, the "deliberate rolling back of public welfare provision and resources, replaced by global corporate commodity chains, has generated profoundly unhealthy community contexts for care" (p. 15). In the AT Clinic featured in chapter four, dignified care emerged locally as physical therapists worked with Hazel and Dean toward a good-enough-for-now wheelchair fit. But consider critical disability scholars' distinction between accommodation and access: "accommodation is usually understood to be an individual, often informal, ad hoc solution to a particular problem, whereas access is meant to provide a structural solution" that is not "reactive and individualized" (Diedrich, 2019, p. 580). Plenty of ad hoc approaches to care exist, and this book seeks not to minimize the enormous impact such projects have had on people's lives. But are these ad hoc solutions sustainable? I worry that within an accommodation, rather than an access, framework, dignified care as ethical praxis could be seen as a sterilized, heroic, or ad hoc version of care that fails to contend with structural injustices.

So, it is important to hold chapter four's conclusions in tension with what Berlant (2004) critiques as the neoliberal practice of "asking individuals and local institutions to take up the obligation to ameliorate the suffering that used to be addressed by the state" (p. 3). Critical health researchers describe how large-scale health care is a neoliberal enterprise, which is a way of indexing how the state assumes a "minimalist role" and reckons that "the market will take care of human, societal, cultural, political, and economic needs" (Dutta, 2016, p. 24). It may be tempting in this neoliberal, market-driven moment to fall back on a form of care that hinges on individualized empathic performances. But as we saw in the

MAiD testimony of chapter three, such an understanding can create conditions wherein some persons' dependency is pathologized while other persons' caretaking is valorized. Logics in popular discourse that warrant some persons' biopolitical in/disposability can and do accrete as forms of eugenicist biopolitical governance. Groenhout (2019) puts it this way: "social structures are not generated or sustained purely by individual decisions, but are instead created and maintained in part by inattention and habit" (p. 13). Through inattention and habit, which enable indifference to difference, individual actions are perpetually prone within, or are susceptible to, an ecology of necropolitical praxis. "They pre-exist the individual and take on a sort of life of their own that is sometimes immune to what individuals would choose if they could" (Groenhout, p. 13). It seems that I cannot, after all, "be the change." What I can do, however, is stay with the trouble by refusing to let myself off the hook.

Given care's complicity with infrastructural harm, Maria Puig de la Casa (2017) attempts to "reclaim care" by acknowledging the "poisons in the grounds that we inhabit rather than expecting to find an outside alternative, untouched by trouble" (p. 11); rather than purging ourselves of or attempting to polish away in/dignity's rough spots (e.g., telling only the first part of the Bill story), we must first consider our "purist ambitions . . . as the utmost poisonous" (p. 11). Similarly, "*harmony*—the absence of outright conflict—often leaves deeper complications untouched" (Brown, 2020, p. 40). In other words, doing dignity does not "erase unresolvable tensions" (Puig de la Casa, p. 11). We must, as Haraway (2016) says, "stay with the trouble." Staying with the trouble involves an ongoing series of self-conscious and trans-corporeal "tinkerings" that never quite "smooth out its asperities" (Puig de la Casa, p. 11). Recall from chapter four the bright-red toolbox always propped open in the center of the AT Clinic. Tinkering is just part of the work of doing dignity. Giraud describes it thus: "Staying with the trouble is intended to resist the 'moral solace' of totalizing ethical imperatives" (p. 122). After all, "moral righteousness is delusional" (Mol, 2021, p. 99). And yet, we cannot let ourselves off the hook.

In chapter seven of her book *I'm Still Here: Black Dignity in a World Made for Whiteness,* Austin Channing Brown (2020) explains what it looks like not to be let off the hook. She was once surrounded after a speaking engagement by white audience members who confessed to her their past racial harms: "Black women were bearing the brunt of these stories as white attenders sought relief from guilt over the ways they had participated in racism. None of them seemed to consider how their confessions affected the people hearing them" (p. 108). Brown affirms that what white people want from so-called reconciliation is "a Black person forgiving them for one racist sin" (p. 110). Recognizing that she cannot make herself "responsible for the transformation of white people," Brown wonders about the possibility of responding to such requests for reconciliation with "So what are you going to do differently?" (p. 110). And that is the question doing dignity asks of us: What are you going to *do* differently?

In her most recent "empirical philosophy" of being, knowing, doing, and relating by way of the deceptively banal practice of eating, Annemarie Mol (2021) writes, "My eating is not a natural, life-affirming endeavor on top of which further ethical commitments may be layered. Instead, my eating is always already technically and socially mediated . . . Moreover, while eating may contribute to my 'vital goodness,' it may also undermine it" (p. 96). Now reread this passage, only this time swap out the words "my eating" with "doing dignity." Doing dignity as ethical praxis insists on practicing iterative rhetorical tasks that are rooted not in an individual's bestowing the "gift" of acknowledgment. In fact, "*doing* eludes the control of a willful center" altogether (Mol, 2021, p. 94). Doing dignity is a multiscalar, trans-corporeal endeavor that "hinges not on decisions and choices, but on trying and adjusting" (Mol, p. 137).

As figure 5.1 illustrates, I see a humbly hopeful future where doing dignity might be therapeutic. Already, forms of so-called dignity therapy have emerged in clinical care contexts in North America and elsewhere. In his book *Dignity Therapy: Final Words for Final Days*, Harvey Chochinov (2012), the originator of "dignity therapy," describes an approach to individual psychotherapy predicated on the model of dignity in the terminally ill. Dignity therapy couples the coauthoring of one's discursive end-of-life legacy with what Chochinov calls "generativity," which he describes as "investing in those who will outlive us" (p. 37). Dignity therapy is an impressive and professionally researched intervention into what in/dignities at the end of life might look like. Although I see opportunities for rhetorically tinkering with the material-discursive methods mobilized by dignity therapy practitioners,[6] the practice is a robust model for the kinds of "thought-reflection-action, and thought-reflection on this action" I am calling for in this chapter (Walsh & Mignolo, 2018, p. 7). Fundamentally, I see dignity therapy as a systematized practice of dignified care that uses qualitative research methods such as semi-structured interviews to *do* dignity. Dignity therapy is but one tangible example of the ways care workers have attempted to marry clinical tasks of caring with the "real time recognition of another's exposure to exposedness" (Davis, 2010, p. 11)—which, in dignity therapy, is one's exposedness to death, or finitude.

On one hand, my presentation of dignity as a practice in this book has relied on analyses of discrete, and markedly different, contexts. On the other hand, such an approach, I hope, has helped readers better understand, through "diverse exemplary situations" (Mol, 2021, p. 20), how in/dignities emerge at different scales. Throughout, I have argued that, while material conditions for ethical praxis are contingent on both scope and situation, there is still a space for human agency. I encourage readers to recalibrate their understanding of in/dignities such that they are always pragmatic, situational, and sensitive to scalar variation—whether one is responding to a global health crisis, a proposed state law, or an intimate clinical encounter. Collectively, the analyses from each chapter have generated conclusions about rhetorical responsivity to stratified livability.

In addition to providing readers with numerous illustrations of how in/dignities both emerge and are enacted, findings from each case study contribute to debates in critical, cultural, and rhetorical theory. Inspired by Wynter's (2003) critique of the "(Western bourgeois) conception of the human, Man," who "overrepresents itself as if it were the human itself" (p. 260), I have grappled with questions about who is, was, or can be regarded as human in the first place. Who gets to decide? And how? *Doing Dignity* suggests that in/dignities emerge concomitantly with non-human things like a contagious airborne virus, the availability of a lethal pharmaceutical cocktail, or the thickness of a wheelchair's seat cushion.

Said simply, the goal of this project has been to suss out actionable tactics for responding to human suffering. I've inquired into the viability of a timeworn, often contradictorily applied, construct—namely, human dignity—as it faces "globalization, technoscience, late capitalism and climate change" (Herbrechter, 2013, p. 94). By illustrating for readers what doing dignity *can* look like in real-time practice, I hope readers might more readily recognize for themselves "possibilities for being otherwise" (Grosz, 2011, p. 14). Eschewing spectacular rhetorics and the "sentimental scripting of hopelessness" (Bargetz, 2019, p. 185), readers might become more sensitive to how dignified care can be cultivated situationally. As an antidote to the "inhuman structures of our times" (Braidotti & Hlavajova, 2018, p. 12), practicing dignified care requires that we continually "start, stop, begin again, but in a different way" (Mol, 2021, p. 142).

APPENDIX A

Corpora Specifications for MAiD Testimony

TABLE A.1.
Summary of data sources

State	Date	Type of data and URL*
Nevada	May 29, 2017, MAiD hearing	SB 261 https://www.leg.state.nv.us/App/NELIS/REL/79th2017/Bill/5197/Overview Minutes and exhibits https://www.leg.state.nv.us/Session/79th2017/Minutes/Assembly/HHS/Final/1287.pdf Audio-visual recording http://sg001-harmony.sliq.net/00324/Harmony/en/PowerBrowser/PowerBrowserV2/20170529/-1/?fk=1858&viewmode=1
	February 25, 2019, MAiD hearing	SB 165 https://www.leg.state.nv.us/App/NELIS/REL/80th2019/Bill/6236/Overview Amendment https://www.leg.state.nv.us/App/NELIS/REL/80th2019/Bill/6236/Text Minutes and exhibits (including written testimony) https://www.leg.state.nv.us/Session/80th2019/Minutes/Senate/HHS/Final/359.pdf Audio-visual recording https://sg001-harmony.sliq.net/00324/Harmony/en/PowerBrowser/PowerBrowserV2/20190225/-1/?fk=173&viewmode=1

(continued)

TABLE A.1.
Continued

State	Date	Type of data and URL*
	April 7, 2021, MAiD hearing	HB 351 https://www.leg.state.nv.us/App/NELIS/REL/81st2021/Bill/7903/Text Minutes and exhibits (including written testimony) https://www.leg.state.nv.us/Session/81st2021/Minutes/Assembly/HHS/Final/789.pdf Audio-visual recording https://sg001-harmony.sliq.net/00324/Harmony/en/PowerBrowser/PowerBrowserV2/20210407/-1/?fk=7995&viewmode=1
Connecticut	February 22, 2021, MAiD hearing	HB 6425 https://www.cga.ct.gov/asp/cgabillstatus/cgabillstatus.asp?selBillType=Bill&bill_num=HB06425&which_year=2021 Written testimony https://www.cga.ct.gov/aspx/CGADisplayTestimonies/CGADisplayTestimony.aspx?bill=HB-06425&doc_year=2021 Audio-visual recording https://www.youtube.com/watch?v=eZgsQorE2sM
	February 17, 2022, MAiD hearing	SB 88 https://www.cga.ct.gov/asp/cgabillstatus/cgabillstatus.asp?selBillType=Bill&bill_num=SB00088&which_year=2022 Written testimony https://www.cga.ct.gov/aspx/CGADisplayTestimonies/CGADisplayTestimony.aspx?bill=SB-00088&doc_year=2022 Audio-visual recording https://www.youtube.com/watch?v=Dsp_ZhQwSJI

* HB = (state) House Bill; SB = (state) Senate Bill

TABLE A.2.

Nevada corpus: MAiD stance of written testimony, by year (n = 60)

Year	Against MAiD	For MAiD
2017	13	9
2019	11	4
2021	4	19
TOTAL	28	32

TABLE A.3.

Nevada corpus: Positionality and stance, by frequency

Positionality	Against MAiD	For MAiD	TOTAL
Clergy	1	0	1
Lawyer or politician	4	4	8
Health care professional	7	6	13
Nonprofit organization or advocacy group	8	9*	17
Resident of the state	9	12	21

* Eight of the nine came from the Compassion & Choices Action Network, a nonprofit from Oregon, which advocates for death-with-dignity laws in states around the country

TABLE A.4.

Connecticut corpus: MAiD stance of written testimony, by year (n = 472)

Year	Against MAiD	For MAiD
2021	116	100
2022	127	129
TOTAL	243	229*

* Excluded was written testimony that replicated prose from Compassion & Choices' sample form letter provided on its website (n = 338 form letters)

TABLE A.5.

Connecticut corpus: Positionality and stance, by frequency

Positionality*	Against MAiD	For MaiD	TOTAL
Clergy	12	7	19
Lawyer or politician	12	14	26
Nonprofit organization or advocacy group	41	18	59
Health care professional	61	44	105
Resident of the state	118	76	194

* Some of those who testified belonged to more than one positionality

APPENDIX B

Inventory of Data from the AT Clinic

TABLE B.1.
Summary of data sources

AT Clinic client	Objects of study
Hazel	140 minutes of video data (plus another 60 minutes of unrecorded/untranscribed observation); approximately 6,000 words of field notes; 15,200 words of transcription data; 6 still images
Dean	63 minutes of video data; approximately 2,000 words of field notes; 10,500 words of transcription data

Chapter 1 · Undoing Dignity

1. The nurse's explanation of the hand-of-God technique was translated into English from Portuguese. I am grateful to Casey Boyle, who thought of my project when he encountered this photograph and shared it with me.

2. A robust discussion of the (neoliberal) relationship among emotion, sympathy, compassion, and empathy can be found in the opening chapter of Berlant's edited collection, where Marjorie Garber (2014) traces the etymology of "compassion." More recently, Groenhout (2019) notes that the very ways in which "social structures" are shaped "sometimes determines what counts as an empathetic response" (p. 13).

3. See, for example, Chávez (2013) and Hesford (2011, 2015, 2021).

4. See Minear (2011).

5. See Jackson (2020).

6. See, for example, Boyle (2018), Edbauer (2005), Gries (2015), Stormer and McGreavy (2017), and Teston (2017a). But also see Madison Jones's (2021) counterhistory of rhetorical ecologies.

7. See Hannah Kihalani Springer's assertion "I am shaped by my geography" (qtd. in Meyer, 2001, p. 128).

8. See also Blake's (2009) *The African Origins of Rhetoric.*

9. See, for example, Debes (2017), Gilabert (2019), Kateb (2011), Killmister (2020), Malpas and Lickiss (2007), McClellan (2019), McCrudden (2013), Muders (2017), Shershow (2014), and Shroeder & Bani-Sadr (2017).

10. In ways I see as aligned with Yergeau, in her summary of Irigaray's and Grosz's emphasis on the corporeal body as a meaningful contributor to a feminist ethic of care, Whatmore (1997) states, "the body is considered not as the passive container of social being but as a living assemblage of biological materials and processes which both register and orient our senses of the world";

furthermore, "such an understanding of the body undermines the political myth of self-authorship and the privileged ethical status of humans as cognitive, communicative subjects" (pp. 43–44).

11. Throughout, when I reference an or the "Other," I'm motivated by Levinas's (1981) (and subsequently Diane Davis's [2005]) conception of "the human Other," or *A/autrui*. I wish not to exclude nonhuman Others, however. Lipari (2014) summarizes Levinas's "other" as a construct in a way quite apt for my purposes: "to make the stranger a familiar is to do violence to the otherness of the other, to exclude some part of the stranger"; instead, she argues (drawing on Levinas), we must not "absorb the other into conformity with the self" but rather create "a dwelling space to receive the alterity of the other and let it resonate" (p. 198).

12. In Boyle's own words, "practice is the exercise of tendencies to activate greater capacities" (p. 5).

13. Saldaña & Omasta (2022) define a case study as "a focused research study on one unit of interest—one person, one setting, one organization, one event, etc." (p. 305). And Blakeslee and Fleischer's (2019) definition provides even more guidance: "Case studies are usually focused on a specific event, activity, or individual within a setting. Case study researchers try to understand that event, activity, or individual in depth, much like ethnographers, but are more interested in the particularities of their single case, rather than the whole culture, although the impact of the culture on the individual might well be considered and/or play a significant role" (p. 99).

14. Throughout, I employ "biopolitical" to emphasize how rhetorical situations are fraught with politics, power differentials, and existential uncertainty. I appreciate Murray's (2022) succinct articulation: "biopolitics is both the medicalization of politics and the politicization of medicine" (p. 23). For a robust critique of the ways "biopolitics" is a whitewashed descriptor for "racialized assemblages," though, see Alexander Weheliye's (2014) *Habeas Viscus*. See also Mbembe's (2019) definition of "biopower": "that domain of life over which power has asserted its control" (p. 66); it is a construct that Mbembe sees as "insufficient" when attempting "to account for contemporary forms of the subjugation of life to the power of death" (p. 92).

15. Instead of "death-with-dignity" or "assisted dying," readers might be more familiar with previously used (now passé) terms such as "euthanasia" or "physician-assisted suicide."

16. In response to this question, I am aligned with Andorno (2009), who notes that "respect for persons is just the *consequence* of human dignity, not dignity itself, in a similar way that the bell's sound is an effect produced by the bell, not the bell itself" (p. 230).

17. For example, Miriam Griffin (2008) postulates that there are "other

Romans more representative than Cicero" when it comes to theorizing human dignity (p. 51).

18. See Van Der Graaf and Van Delden (2009, p. 153).

19. See also Pico della Mirandola's *De hominis dignitate* of 1486 and the US Supreme Court's recent decision to overturn the precedent set by the decision in *Roe v. Wade.*

20. But again, see Debes's (2017) *Dignity: A History* for alternative historical accounts.

21. There is debate about whether Kantian dignity is really all that different from Greco-Roman notions of dignity based on status. I tend to agree with Formosa (2017), who argues that Kantian ethics tries to have it both ways; that is, Kantian dignity is both rank-based *and* value-based: "This is because the status or rank that persons have for the Kantian is that of possessing absolute worth or dignity" (p. 7).

22. Jurgen Habermas (2010) argues that human dignity, even within a rights-based framework, still depends on status and rank—specifically, the "status of democratic citizenship" (p. 464).

23. See also Evelin Lindner's (2001) work on humiliation.

24. Here I'm influenced by Lisa Diedrich's (2019) assertion that human vulnerability is "a condition that a rights framework often fails to account for or remedy adequately" (p. 574). See also Jasbir Puar (2017).

25. I want to quote at length Astrida Neimanis (2017), who summarizes this groundbreaking work well and with plenty of in-text citations, to boot:

> . . . there is a pressing need to acknowledge feminist, anticolonial, and queer thinking more generally as facilitating much of our "new" ecological thinking, and "new" materialisms particularly (see Ahmed 2008; Sullivan 2012). For four decades, ecofeminism in particular (e.g. Gaard 1993; Kheel 1993; Warren 1997) has been encouraging us to recognize the connections between the derogation of certain kinds of human bodies, and a mistreatment of environmental bodies, including other animals; queer feminisms (e.g. Ahmed 2006; Chen 2012; Gaard 1997; Sandilands 2001; Seymour 2013) have asked us to pay attention to those bodies—both human and more-than-human—which challenge teleological norms and straight stories of proliferation and fecundity; anticolonial feminisms have asked us to resist human exceptionalism in our valuations of worlds that sustain us—which connects strongly to feminist approaches to environmental justice that argue that when it comes to intercorporeal vulnerabilities, some skins are more porous than others (e.g. Andrea Smith 1997; LaDuke 1999). Some versions of feminist technoscience studies have encouraged more critical and creative views of the matters that corporeally make us and connect us (see Åsberg 2013).

Black feminisms, and other women of colour feminisms, above all, have taught us about difference—as a prerequisite for justice, and as a source of empowerment and strength (see Anzaldua 1987; hooks 2000; Lorde 1984). (pp. 8–9)

26. See also Nirmala Erevelles (2011). But note, too, that "Haraway is keenly aware of the tendency to erase racial histories; to claim a post racial moment as a way of erasing the ongoing violence and historic trauma of racial Western history" (Adams & Weinstein, 2020, p. 236).

27. Asberg, Thiele, and van der Tuin (2015) describe materialist feminist scholarship (which is adjacent to and at times overlaps with critical feminist posthumanism) this way: "For materialist feminist scholars, trained with a political pathos that taps into sexual difference, feminist science studies, anti-colonial, environmental, animal and social justice movements, we certainly can agree with the need to acknowledge the nonhuman (poor term, of course) agentiality." They continue: "Yet we cannot help but wonder what happened to connectivity, power-imbued codependencies and what, for example, feminist environmental scholar Stacy Alaimo (2016) calls the 'trans-corporeal'—describing the movement across human embodiment and nonhuman nature—and other similar concepts for the *formative topologies of force and power* that cause us to materialize" (pp. 148–149; emphasis added).

Chapter 2 · COVID-19 Caretaking

1. "We typically use three team members on either side of the patient and respiratory at the head of the bed to manage the patient's airway. We then gently and strategically roll them from their back to side and then prone on the stomach" (*Art of Proning*, 2021). This 45-second video demonstrates the complexity of proning a patient: https://twitter.com/MEDspirationNFP/status/1432706393027588109?s=20&t=d11oC2Xc-d539OIMDKSkzw.

2. Throughout, I'm using Barad's (2007) notion of "apparatus," which is a generic referent for the sociopolitical, material-discursive condition(alitie)s that intra-act over time to co-constitute what we call phenomena. See her interview in Juelskjær and Schwennesen (2012) for a more detailed account of what she means by "apparatus," especially page 11.

3. Hendren (2020) points out how infrastructures, because of their ubiquity, go "to sleep in our consciousness" (p. 201). This is what I'm alluding to by using the word "aside."

4. The notion of the "double bind" first proposed by Gregory Bateson et al. (1956) and, later, picked up by Gayatri Chakravorty Spivak (2012) may also be helpful here for understanding how "particular, localized, and phenomenologi-

cal experiences" exist concomitantly with "institutional structures," such as "capitalism, racism, ableism, the law, medicine, family, etc." (Diedrich, 2019, p. 575).

5. Here I wonder whether this is what Mbembe (2019) means by "zero world" (p. 167).

6. The research for this first case study was approved by Ohio State University's institutional review board (protocol #2020B0264) and was sponsored by Ohio State University's Global Arts + Humanities Discovery Theme.

7. I am grateful to Victoria Charoonratana, MD, and Lauren Terbrock-Elmestad, PhD, for their assistance with this pilot study, which was originally (before COVID-19) focused on how early-career HCPs perceived and practiced human dignity.

8. I have no doubt that volunteer bias played a significant part in the forthcoming analyses. That is, the HCPs who volunteered to participate likely had some type of motivation—however implicit—to tell a story about their COVID-19 caretaking experiences. The "opt-in" nature of participant recruitment for this study affects findings. Nevertheless, participants' narratives, regardless of what motivated their decision to share them, provide a meaningful record of one of the most challenging moments in US (and global) health care.

9. For more on the productive power of (dis)orientation, see Sarah Ahmed's (2006) *Queer Phenomenology*.

10. Anna Tsing et al.'s (2021) *Feral Atlas* highlights what she calls "tippers" as one of three analytic axes for understanding climate catastrophe. Throughout, when I refer to "infrastructures," I'm inspired by Tsing's notion of tippers, which are otherwise mundane if not deceptively small "non-designed effects" on large-scale systems. Such non-designed effects can be catastrophic: "It's not just that atmospheric carbon dioxide increases; at some point that increase starts to have systems-changing effects, which in turn will affect most life on earth" (n.p.). The infrastructural failures part of HCPs' caretaking inheritances were predicated on a host of tippers' non-designed effects.

11. See Blum's (2019) chapter in *The Ethics of Care* for an interesting discussion of guilt and care as "repaying the debt" (p. 10).

12. Many of these biases were rooted in some of the larger biopolitical topoi I'll go on to describe in the next chapter.

13. I'm thinking here, too, of Hill's (2002) notion of the "kairotic happening," which includes "single events containing multiple ones." Each kairotic event is "an instantaneous now that embeds the whole episode. Every circumstance has its own continually transforming moments that resonate with others, so kairotic openings are indeed points of present time tied to all other moments, past and present, which have unfolded qualitatively in the time of this situation" (p. 216).

Chapter 3 · *Death-with-Dignity's Biopolitical* Topoi

1. I'm uneasy about whether to call MAiD hearings "deliberative" since, after spending months if not years with these data, participants' testimony embodies "what epideictic rhetoric is all about: a desire for truth; a willingness to open oneself to what *is*; the courage to confess, to admit publicly one's worldview; and the skill to present this confession in an appropriate and thus fitting manner to others who wait for their interests to be acknowledged" (Hyde, 2006, p. 79).

2. This quotation and others from testimonies at state hearings came from my Connecticut and Nevada corpora. See appendix A for information about these sources and their availability.

3. For more detail about MAiD's legal history, see Pope (2018).

4. For more on "decision-making capacity," see Simplican's (2015) *The Capacity Contract: Intellectual Disability and the Question of Citizenship.*

5. See, for example, Barton (2005), Barton et al. (2005), Cain and McCleskey (2019), Grim (2005), Kopelson 2019.

6. See Barton (2005) for more on how infrequently advance directives were relied on, at least in 2005, when discussing end of life matters.

7. I am enormously grateful to Rheanna Velasquez and Olivia Andresen for their tireless labor and for Ohio State University's College of Arts & Sciences Completion Grant, which financially supported this project.

8. According to Public Policy Polling, 72% of Nevada voters support MAiD. According to Greenberg Quinian Rosner, 75% of Connecticut voters support MAiD. For a summary of these poll results and others, see Compassion & Choices (2022, pp. 9–10, 4–5).

9. I decided to exclude written testimony that replicated prose from Compassion & Choices' form letter provided on its website. My rationale for this exclusion was rooted in a desire to understand how Connecticut residents reasoned about and mobilized evidence in making arguments about MAiD—in their own words—not in a desire to quantify how many people wrote in favor of or against MAiD legislation.

10. By "both sides of the MAiD debate," I am oversimplifying for the purpose of readability. There was a third stance on MAiD: the neutral stance. Only six forms of written testimony took the neutral stance; such a stance was taken by representatives of relevant nonprofit organizations who participated in the hearing to offer expertise on the matter, either in the form of improving some of the bill's language or to add nuance to some of the bill's particulars.

11. Word search queries in NVivo for "mom/mother" and "dad/father" indicated that these terms appeared almost equally across the two stances.

12. For more on the ways that logics of choice are distinct from care-in-practice, see Annemarie Mol (2008).

13. Barton's (2005) results point toward the complexity of control or autonomy in North American medicine. More particularly, it's not that "decisions" are made at the end of life; it's that parties are involved in building consensus.

14. Eschewing the assumed distinction between bodies and minds, Margaret Price (2015) proposes a "crip politics of bodyminds" (p. 269).

15. For more on the harms of ventriloquizing at the end of life, see Hansen (2012).

16. Not only were these forms of testimony persuasive to me, but such testimony also resulted in state representatives choosing to ask follow-up questions after the testimony was complete. Follow-up questions from state representatives happened so infrequently that it signified to me that something about the testimony had piqued their interest.

17. When Mr. Gillums granted me permission to reveal his identity, he reminded me that while he was an executive of the National Alliance on Mental Illness (NAMI) at the time of the hearing, he "did not / could not state an organizational position as a NAMI spokesperson as NAMI does not weigh in on such issues" (personal email communication, 6/6/2022).

Chapter 4 · Embodied Dignities in an Assistive Technology

1. The research for this case study was approved by Ohio State University's institutional review board (protocol #2016B0361).

2. Micro-moment, as an analytical construct, is also informed by Hindmarsh and Pilnick's (2002) description of each element of an interaction as "context shaped and context renewing, both organized in the light of the prior action and framing the next" (p. 143).

3. From this point on, when I discuss "conditions," I'm invoking an Arendtian sense of conditionality—*vita activa*—which indexes how "human existence" is "comprised of a constellation of conditions" (Macready, 2018, p. 30); in this sense, conditions both "make something possible" and are the result of "the gathering of those conditions" (pp. 18–19). I can't help but understand Arendtian conditionality through the prism of co-production or co-constitution (Teston, 2018, p. 11) as well as Alaimo's (2018) notion of trans-corporeality.

4. See also Hird (2004) and Willey (2016).

5. Karen Barad (2007) might refer to these dynamic relationships as a series of "intra-actions."

6. For another rhetorical take on "fit," readers might be interested in S. Scott Graham's (2020) *Where's the Rhetoric?* wherein he, channeling Alfred North Whitehead, describes fit in terms of "satisfaction" (pp. 73–75).

7. See the Land Grab U project at https://www.landgrabu.org/.

8. In accordance with privacy assurances required by the institutional review board, the physical therapists working at the AT Clinic agreed to screen and invite patients who met my study's eligibility criteria.

9. I struggled with deciding what to call these data: stories, narratives, or a socially scientific series of observations? In the end, I settled on a hybrid approach that I hope honors the humanity of my participants and remains vigilant to the ways that storytelling from my own limited positionality might color my representations of participants' experiences. I hope readers will understand the ethnographic difficulty associated with telling a compelling story while respecting that some stories are not mine to tell. I worry very much about being or becoming what Scuro (2017) terms "the ablebodied interloper" (p. xxxii). I'm also extremely mindful of what Svendby, Romsland, and Moen (2018) have described as "non-disabled ableism," which risks, as Garland-Thomson (2009) says, "reproducing a pattern in which disabled people are yet again exotified through a non-disabled gaze, or even a 'non-disabled stare'" (p. 222).

10. At no time did I have access to Hazel's medical record; rather, her physical therapist, Stephanie, read abbreviated excerpts from it during one of her appointments to inform the wheelchair vendor about Hazel's needs.

11. Sara Hendren (2020) describes how "assistive technologies" as a phrase is redundant (p. 25).

12. By the time I received institutional approval to observe AT Clinic sessions, Hazel had already met with the AT Clinic physician to discuss her mobility needs and had a preliminary meeting with Stephanie. Therefore, what I'm calling Hazel's first appointment was actually her third appointment at the AT Clinic.

13. Williamson (2019) provides historical context for how post–World War II spaces for physical therapy and rehabilitation were designed to include simulation technologies.

14. Because of how it ultimately shaped my findings, grounded theorists would call "contingency" a "sensitizing concept."

15. Grounded theorists would refer to this list as "open codes."

16. Here, once again, I'm influenced by Allen's (2018) discussion of negotiating constraints, which is "a matter of creatively encountering the limits within and of our environments, selves, and others" (p. 259).

17. It wasn't until I read Rowntree's (2019) expert summary of Davis's apt illustration of "exposure to exposedness" that I truly understood its importance in the AT Clinic. Here's Rowntree:

> To illustrate this rhetoricity, Davis picks up [Jean Luc] Nancy's example of exposure and finitude by imagining passengers traveling together on

> a train. The passengers sit in their seats, reading or sleeping or listening to music. They are linked by location and the temporal juncture of being together in the same space at the same time, even along the same trajectory; however, as a singularity of being-with, they are "nothing but this suspension between disintegration and aggregation" (9). They are not yet a community, for "indifference is the luxury of exposed existents who are not faced with the fact of their exposedness" (10). The passengers are gathered and exposed to danger and mortality, but they are not aware nor are they attending to the material conditions of those around them. The passengers do not need to face their exposure until something happens—a wreck, a terrorist attack, or some other disaster. The disaster prompts a sudden realization of their exposure to finitude that brings the passengers face-to-face. (p. 52)

18. Ellingson (2017) describes in detail how "verbal and nonverbal communication choices form part of a horizontal web (or mesh, or nexus, or net) of practices that hang together. The practices in which they (bodily) engage come to constitute situated meanings of . . . care giving and care receiving" (p. 13).

19. In the parlance of grounded theory, these are "axial codes."

20. Grounded theory would term these four practices "selective codes."

21. See Bess Williamson's (2019) *Accessible America*, which devotes an entire chapter to discussing the politics of wheelchair ramps. Her argument is premised on the assertion that "the claims for a seamless 'design for all' conceal the inequalities embedded in design and space themselves" (p. 13)—an argument that adds another dimension to why it's important to be sensitive to "varying vulnerability" (Niccolini & Ringrose, 2019, p. 2).

22. Hazel and Dean were asked to rank, on a scale of 1–10, their pain levels when performing a simulation. They were also asked to rank, on a scale of 1–10, how difficult they felt it was to operate the wheelchair when performing a simulation.

23. See Remi Yergeau's (2018) reworking, or cripping and queering, of rhetoricity to account for a/symbolic "ecophenomena" (p. 179).

24. Readers who aren't pianists may not be familiar with how different the weight of a keyboard's keys feel under a pianist's fingertips when compared to the weight of a piano's keys. Some pianists refer to this weighted feeling as an instrument's "action." It's difficult to describe the differences in feel, but they're significant to those of us who play the piano.

Chapter 5 · Dignified Care as Ethical Praxis

1. As Nikolas Rose (2009) concludes in *The Politics of Life Itself: Biomedicine, Power, and Subjectivity in the Twenty-First Century*, modern-day health care can

embody "cynicism, pragmatism, ambition, greed, and rivalry," but, he argues, it is "also inescapably searching for, assembling, and inventing ways in which they [participants in the health care system] might evaluate, adjudicate, and ethically justify the decisions they must make when human vitality is at stake" (p. 257). Doing dignity requires a similar inescapable "searching for, assembling, and inventing"—a doing that is never done.

2. Among the other types of dignity that Jacobson (2012) describes are personal dignity, comportment dignity, dignity-of-self, dignity-in-relation, adverbial dignity, and collective dignity (pp. 14–17).

3. See, for example, Condit (2008), Happe (2013), Davis (1983), Fixmer-Oraiz (2019), Kluchin (2011), Koerber (2018), Nelson (2003), Roberts (1997), Ross (2017), Rusert (2012), TallBear (2013), Theobold (2019), Washington (2006), and Yam (2020).

4. See also McKittrick's (2015) *Sylvia Wynter: On Being Human as Praxis.*

5. See also Fox's (1983) "Ancient Egyptian Rhetoric."

6. In fact, Chochinov (2012) says that the practice he advocates is rooted in Rogerian rhetoric (or what's called "client-centered therapy" in psychology).

REFERENCES

Adams, J. D., & Weinstein, M. (2020). Sylvia Wynter: Science studies and posthumanism as praxes of being human. *Cultural Studies ↔ Critical Methodologies, 20*(3), 235–250.

Ahmed, S. (2006). *Queer phenomenology: Orientations, objects, others.* Duke University Press.

Ahmed, S. (2014). *The cultural politics of emotion.* Edinburgh University Press.

Alaimo, S. (2008). Trans-corporeal feminisms and the ethical space of nature. *Material Feminisms, 25*(2), 237–264.

Alaimo, S. (2016). *Exposed: Environmental politics and pleasures in posthuman times.* University of Minnesota Press.

Alaimo, S. (2018). Trans-corporeality. *Posthuman glossary* (pp. 435–438). Bloomsbury.

Allen, I. (2018). *The ethical fantasy of rhetorical theory.* University of Pittsburgh Press.

Aluli-Meyer, M. (2013). Indigenous and authentic: Hawaiian epistemology and the triangulation of meaning. In M. K. Asante, Y. Miike, & J. Yin (Eds.), *The global intercultural communication reader* (pp. 148–164). Routledge.

Andorno, R. (2009). Human dignity and human rights as a common ground for a global bioethics. *Journal of Medicine and Philosophy, 34,* 223–240.

Antonovich, J. (2021). White coats, white hoods: The medical politics of the Ku Klux Klan in 1920s America. *Bulletin of the History of Medicine, 95*(4), 437–463.

Arendt, H. (2013). *The human condition.* University of Chicago Press (Original work published in 1958).

The art of proning. (2021). Johns Hopkins Medicine. https://www.hopkinsmedicine.org/news/articles/the-art-of-proning

Asberg, C., Thiele, K., & van der Tuin, I. (2015). Speculative before the turn: Reintroducing feminist materialist performativity. *Cultural Studies Review, 21*(2), 145–172.

Asen, R. (2010). Reflections on the role of rhetoric in public policy. *Rhetoric and Public Affairs, 13*(1), 121–143.

Barad, K. (2003). Posthumanist performativity: Toward an understanding of how matter comes to matter. *Signs: Journal of Women in Culture and Society, 28*(3), 801–831.

Barad, K. (2007). *Meeting the universe halfway: Quantum physics and the entanglement of matter and meaning.* Duke University Press.

Barad, K. (2012). On touching—the inhuman that therefore I am. *differences, 23*(3), 206–223.

Bargetz, B. (2019). Longing for agency: New materialisms' wrestling with despair. *European Journal of Women's Studies, 26*(2), 181–194.

Barton, E. (2005). Institutional policies, professional practices, and the discourse of end-of-life discussions in American medicine. *Journal of Applied Linguistics, 2*(3), 253–271.

Barton, E. (2007). Situating end-of-life decision making in a hybrid ethical frame. *Communication and Medicine, 4*(2), 131–140.

Barton, E., Aldridge, M., Trimble, T., & Vidovik, J. (2005). Structure and variation in end-of-life discussion in American medicine. *Communication & Medicine, 2,* 3–20.

Basu, A., & Dutta, M. J. (2007). Centralizing context and culture in the co-construction of health: Localizing and vocalizing health meanings in rural India. *Health Communication, 21*(2), 187–196.

Bateson, G., Jackson, D. D., Haley, J., & Weakland, John. (1956). Toward a theory of schizophrenia. *Behavioral Science, 1*(4), 251–264.

Battin, M. P. (2005). *Ending life: Ethics and the way we die.* Oxford University Press.

Belser, J. W. (2016). Vital wheels: Disability, relationality, and the queer animacy of vibrant things. *Hypatia, 13*(1), pp. 5–21.

Benjamin, R. (2016). Informed refusal: Toward a justice-based bioethics. *Science, Technology, & Human Values, 41*(6), 967–990.

Berghs, M. (2017). Practices and discourses of *ubuntu*: Implications for an African model of disability? *African Journal of Disability, 6*(1), 1–8.

Berlant, L. (2004). *Compassion: The culture and politics of an emotion.* Routledge.

Berlant, L. (2007). Slow death (sovereignty, obesity, lateral agency). *Critical Inquiry, 33*(4), 754–780.

Blake, C. (2010). *The African origins of rhetoric.* Routledge.

Blakeslee, A., & Fleischer, C. (2009). *Becoming a writing researcher.* Routledge.

Blum, A. (2019). Introduction: The dialectic of care. In A. Blum & S. J. Murray (Eds.), *The ethics of care: Moral knowledge, communication, and the art of caregiving* (pp. 1–24). Routledge.

Boyle, C. (2018). *Rhetoric as a posthuman practice.* Ohio State University Press.

Braidotti, R. (2020). "We" are in *this* together, but we are not one and the same. *Journal of Bioethical Inquiry, 17*(4), 465–469.

Braidotti, R., & Hlavajova, M. (Eds.). (2018). Introduction. *Posthuman glossary*. Bloomsbury.

Braswell, H. (2011). Can there be a disability studies theory of "end-of-life autonomy"? *Disability Studies Quarterly, 31*(4). https://dsq-sds.org/article/view/1704/1754

Brezina, V. (2018). Collocation graphs and networks: Selected applications. In P. Cantos-Gómez & M. Almela-Sánchez (Eds.), *Lexical collocation analysis*. Springer.

Brezina, V., Weill-Tessier, P., & McEnery, A. (2020). #LancsBox, version 5.x [Software]. http://corpora.lancs.ac.uk/lancsbox

Brouwer, J., & van Tuinen, S. (Eds.). (2019). *To mind is to care*. V2 Publishing.

Brown, A. C. (2020). *I'm still here: Black dignity in a world made for whiteness*. Hachette UK.

Butchart, G. C. (2019). *Embodiment, relation, community: A continental philosophy of communication*. Penn State University Press.

Cain, C. K., & McCleskey, S. (2019). Expanded definitions of the "good death"? Race, ethnicity and medical aid in dying. *Sociology of Health & Illness, 41*(6), 1175–1191.

Calhoun, D. H. (2013). Human exceptionalism and *imago dei*: The tradition of human dignity. *Human dignity in bioethics: From worldviews to the public square* (pp. 20–45). Routledge.

Campbell, C. S. (2018). Medical aid in dying: Bioethics as sideshow. *Hastings Center Report, 48*(6).

Care Collective. (2020). *The care manifesto*. Verso Books.

Caulfield, T., & Chapman, A. (2005). Human dignity as a criterion for science policy. *PLOS Medicine, 2*, 736–738.

Centers for Disease Control and Prevention. (2022). Nearly one in five American adults who have had COVID-19 still have "long COVID." https://www.cdc.gov/nchs/pressroom/nchs_press_releases/2022/20220622.htm

Chávez, K. R. (2013). *Queer migration politics: Activist rhetoric and coalitional possibilities*. University of Illinois Press.

Chochinov, H. M. (2012). *Dignity therapy: Final words for final days*. Oxford University Press.

Clare, E. (2017). *Brilliant imperfection: Grappling with cure*. Duke University Press.

Colebrook, C. (2020). The future is already deterritorialized. In R. Harrison & C. Sterling (Eds.), *Deterritorializing the future: Heritage in, of and after the Anthropocene* (pp. 346–383). Open Humanities Press.

Compassion & Choices (2022, November 3). *Polling on voter support for medical aid in dying*. https://www.compassionandchoices.org/docs/default-source/fact-sheets/fs---medical-aid-in-dying-survey-results-updated-2.24.22.pdf?sfvrsn=3dc7c5c_1

Condit, C. M. (2008). Race and genetics from a modal materialist perspective. *Quarterly Journal of Speech, 94*(4), 383–406.

Darwall, S. (2017). Equal dignity and rights. In R. Debes (Ed.), *Dignity: A History* (pp. 181–201). Oxford University Press.

Davis, A. (1983). *Women, race, & class*. Knopf Doubleday.

Davis, D. (2005). Addressing alterity: Rhetoric, hermeneutics, and the non-appropriative relation. *Philosophy and Rhetoric, 38*(3), 191–212.

Davis, D. (2010). *Inessential solidarity*. University of Pittsburgh Press.

Davis, D. (2017). Rhetoricity at the end of the world. *Philosophy and Rhetoric, 50*, 431–451.

Death with dignity: An inquiry into related public issues. (1972). US Government Printing Office.

DeathWithDignity.org. (n.d.). News [Hyperlinked news articles listed in descending chronological order]. https://deathwithdignity.org/news/

Debes, R. (Ed.). (2017). *Dignity: A history*. Oxford University Press.

Deloria, V., Deloria Jr., V., & Wildcat, D. (2001). *Power and place: Indian education in America*. Fulcrum Publishing.

De Souza, R. (2009). Creating "communicative spaces": A case of NGO community organizing for HIV/AIDS prevention. *Health Communication, 24*(8), 692–702.

Diedrich, L. (2019). Articulating double binds: Between a rhetoricity of rights and vulnerabilities (relation, pedagogy, care). *South Atlantic Quarterly, 118*(3), 573–594.

Dolmage, J., & Lewiecki-Wilson, C. (2010). Refiguring rhetorica: Linking feminist rhetoric and disability studies. *Rhetorica in motion: Feminist rhetorical methods and methodologies* (pp. 23–38). University of Pittsburgh Press.

Donnelly, J. (1982). Human rights and human dignity: An analytic critique of non-Western conceptions of human rights. *American Political Science Review, 76*(2), 303–316.

Douglass, P. D. (2018). Black feminist theory for the dead and dying. *Theory & Event, 21*(1), 106–123.

Dudley, R. (2012). Toward an understanding of the "medical plantation" as a cultural location of disability. *Disability Studies Quarterly, 32*(4). https://doi.org/10.18061/dsq.v32i4.3248

Dutta, M. J. (2016). *Neoliberal health organizing: Communication, meaning, and politics*. Routledge.

Dutta-Bergman, M. (2005). Theory and practice in health communication campaigns: A critical interrogation. *Health Communication, 18*, 103–122.

Edbauer, J. (2005). Unframing models of public distribution: From rhetorical situation to rhetorical ecologies. *Rhetoric Society Quarterly, 35*(4), 5–24.

Erevelles, N. (2011). *Disability and difference in global contexts: Enabling a transformative body politic.* Palgrave Macmillan.

Fairclough, N. (2013). Critical discourse analysis and critical policy studies. *Critical Policy Studies, 7*, 177–197.

Ferreira da Silva, D. (2018). Hacking the subject: Black feminism and refusal beyond the limits of critique. *PhiloSOPHIA, 8*(1), 19–41.

Fixmer-Oraiz, N. (2019). *Homeland maternity: US security culture and the new reproductive regime.* University of Illinois Press.

Formosa, P. (2017). *Kantian ethics, dignity and perfection.* Cambridge University Press.

Fox, M. V. (1983). Ancient Egyptian rhetoric. *Rhetorica, 1*(1), 9–22.

Fukuyama, F. (2019). *Identity: Contemporary identity politics and the struggle for recognition.* Profile Books.

Fullagar, S., & Pavlidis, A. (2021). Thinking through the disruptive effects and affects of the coronavirus with feminist new materialism. *Leisure Sciences, 43*(1–2), 152–159.

Garber, M. (2014). Compassion. In L. Berlant (Ed.), *Compassion: The culture and politics of an emotion.* Routledge.

Garland-Thomson, R. (1997). *Extraordinary bodies: Figuring disability in American culture and literature.* Columbia University Press.

Garland-Thomson, R. (2017a). Eugenic world building and disability: The strange world of Kazuo Ishiguro's *Never Let Me Go. Journal of Medical Humanities, 38*(2), 133–145.

Garland-Thomson, R. (2017b). Disability bioethics: From theory to practice. *Kennedy Institute of Ethics Journal, 27*(2), 323–339.

Gilabert, P. (2019). *Human dignity and social justice.* Oxford University Press.

Giraud, E. H. (2019). *What comes after entanglement? Activism, anthropocentrism, and an ethics of exclusion.* Duke University Press.

Graham, S. S. (2015). *The politics of pain medicine.* University of Chicago Press.

Graham, S. S. (2020). *Where's the rhetoric? Imagining a unified field.* Ohio State University Press.

Gries, L. (2015). *Still life with rhetoric: A new materialist approach for visual rhetorics.* University Press of Colorado.

Griffin, M. (2017). Dignity in Roman and Stoic thought. In R. Debes (Ed.), *Dignity: A history* (pp. 47–66). Oxford University Press.

Grim, A. (2005). *Citizens deliberate the "good death": The vernacular rhetoric of euthanasia* [Unpublished doctoral dissertation]. University of Colorado at Boulder.

Groenhout, R. E. (2019). *Care ethics and social structures in medicine.* Routledge.

Gröndahl, M., Jacobs, A., & Buchanan, L. (2020, May 8). In the fight to treat coronavirus, your lungs are a battlefield. *New York Times*. https://www.nytimes.com/interactive/2020/05/08/health/coronavirus-covid-lungs-ventilators.html

Gross, A. G., & Dearin, R. D. (2002). *Chaim Perelman*. Southern Illinois University Press.

Grosz, E. (2011). *Becoming undone: Darwinian reflections on life, politics, and art*. Duke University Press.

Gupta, K. (2020). *Medical entanglements: Rethinking feminist debates about healthcare*. Rutgers University Press.

Habermas, J. (2010). The concept of human dignity and the realistic utopia of human rights. *Metaphilosophy, 41*(4), 464–480.

Hamraie, A. (2017). *Building access: Universal design and the politics of disability*. University of Minnesota Press.

"Hand of God": Moving photo of nurse trying to comfort isolated patient in Brazil's Covid ward goes viral. (2021, April 11). *Indian Express*. https://indianexpress.com/article/trending/trending-globally/brazil-nurse-gloves-hand-to-comfort-covid-patient-goes-viral-7265937/.

Hansen, S. (2012). Terri Shiavo and the language of biopolitics. *International Journal of Feminist Approaches to Bioethics, 5*(1), 91–112.

Happe, K. E. (2013). The body of race: Toward a rhetorical understanding of racial ideology. *Quarterly Journal of Speech, 99*(2), 131–155.

Haraway, D. J. (2016). *Staying with the trouble: Making kin in the Chthulucene*. Duke University Press.

Hauser, G. A. (2007). Vernacular discourse and the epistemic dimension of public opinion. *Communication Theory, 17*(4), 333–339.

Heard, M. M. (2013). Tonality and *ethos*. *Philosophy & Rhetoric, 46*(1), 44–64.

Hendren, S. (2020). *What can a body do? How we meet the built world*. Penguin.

Herbrechter, S. (2013). *Posthumanism: A critical analysis*. A & C Black.

Hesford, W. (2011). *Spectacular rhetorics*. Duke University Press.

Hesford, W. S. (2015). Surviving recognition and racial in/justice. *Philosophy & Rhetoric, 48*(4), 536–560.

Hesford, W. S. (2021). *Violent exceptions: Children's human rights and humanitarian rhetorics*. Ohio State University Press.

Hill, A. (2016). Breast cancer's rhetoricity: Bodily border crisis and bridge to corporeal solidarity. *Review of Communication, 16*(4), 281–298.

Hill, C. E. (2002). Changing times in composition classes: *Kairos*, resonance, and the Pythagorean connection. In P. Sipiora & J. S. Baumlin (Eds.), *Rhetoric and kairos: Essays in history, theory, and praxis* (pp. 211–225). State University of New York Press.

Hindmarsh, J., & Pilnick, A. (2002). The tacit order of teamwork: Collaboration and embodied conduct in anesthesia. *Sociological Quarterly, 43*(2), 139–164.

Hird, M. J. (2004). *Sex, gender, and science.* New York: Palgrave.

Ho, A. (2011). Trusting experts and epistemic humility in disability. *IJFAB: International Journal of Feminist Approaches to Bioethics, 4*(2), 102–123.

Hseih, H. F., & Shannon, S. E. (2005). Three approaches to qualitative content analysis. *Qualitative Health Research, 15*(9), 1277–1288.

Hulme, M., & Truch, A. (2005). The role of interspace in sustaining identity. In P. Glotz, S. Berscht, & C. Locke (Eds.), *Thumb culture: The meaning of mobile phones for society.* Transaction Books.

Human dignity and bioethics: Essays commissioned by the President's Council on Bioethics (2008). Government Printing Office.

Hyde, M. J. (2001a). Defining "human dignity" in the debate over the (im)morality of physician-assisted suicide. *Journal of Medical Humanities, 22*(1), 69–82.

Hyde, M. J. (2001b). *The call of conscience: Heidegger and Levinas, rhetoric and the euthanasia debate.* University of South Carolina Press.

Hyde, M. J. (2006). *Life giving gift of acknowledgment.* Purdue University Press.

Hyde, M. J., & McSpiritt, S. (2007). Coming to terms with perfection: The case of Terri Schiavo. *Quarterly Journal of Speech, 93*(2), 150–178.

"I don't want to wake up anymore"—constituent stories inspire Senator Haskell to co-sponsor dignity in dying. (2021, February 26). Connecticut State Democrats [Press release]. http://www.senatedems.ct.gov/haskell-news/3573-haskell-210226#sthash.yPW2OYYp.dpbs

Jackson, Z. I. (2016). Sense of things. *Catalyst: Feminism, Theory, Technoscience, 2*(2), 1–48.

Jackson, Z. I. (2020). *Becoming human.* New York University Press.

Jacobson, N. (2012). *Dignity and health.* Vanderbilt University Press.

Jennings, P. K., & Talley, C. R. (2003). A good death? White privilege and public opinion: Research on euthanasia. *Race, Gender & Class, 10*(3), 42–63.

Jensen, R. E. (2015). An ecological turn in rhetoric of health scholarship: Attending to the historical flow and percolation of ideas, assumptions, and arguments. *Communication Quarterly, 63*(5), 522–526.

Johnson, H. M. (2020). Unspeakable conversations. In A. Wong (Ed.), *Disability visibility: First-person stories from the twenty-first century* (pp. 3–27.). Vintage.

Jones, M. (2021). A counterhistory of rhetorical ecologies. *Rhetoric Society Quarterly, 51*(4), 336–352.

Juelskjær, M., & Schwennesen, N. (2012). Intra-active entanglements—an interview with Karen Barad. *Kvinder, Køn & Forskning, 1–2*, 10–23.

Kafer, A. (2013). *Feminist, queer, crip.* Indiana University Press.

Kafer, A. (2019). Crip kin, manifesting. *Catalyst: Feminism, Theory, Technoscience, 5*(1), 1–37.

Kamwangamalu, N. M. (2013). *Ubuntu* in South Africa: A sociolinguistic perspective to a pan-African concept. *The Global Intercultural Communication Reader.* Routledge.

Karenga, J. (2013). *Nommo, kawaida,* and communicative practice: Bringing good into the world. In M. K. Asante, Y. Miike, & J. Yin (Eds.), *The global intercultural communication reader* (pp. 211–225). Routledge.

Karera, A. (2019). Blackness and the pitfalls of Anthropocene ethics. *Critical Philosophy of Race, 7*(1), 32–56.

Kateb, G. (2011). *Human dignity.* Harvard University Press.

Kenny, R. W. (2005) A cycle of terms implicit in the idea of medicine: Karen Ann Quinlan as a rhetorical icon and the transvaluation of the ethics of euthanasia. *Health Communication, 17*(1), 17–39.

Keränen, L. (2007). "'Cause someday we all die": Rhetoric, agency, and the case of the "patient" preferences worksheet. *Quarterly Journal of Speech, 93*(2), 179–210.

Killmister, S. (2020). *Contours of dignity.* Oxford University Press.

King, T. L. (2017). Humans involved: Lurking in the lines of posthumanist flight. *Critical Ethnic Studies, 3*(1), 162–185.

Kittay, E. F. (2005). Equality, dignity, and disability. In M. A. Lyons & F. Waldron (Eds.), *Perspectives on equality: The second Seamus Heaney lectures.* Liffey Press.

Klamer, A. (2019). The battle of cares. In J. Brouwer & S. van Tuinen (Eds.), *To mind is to care* (pp. 174–188). V2 Publishing.

Kluchin, R. M. (2011). *Fit to be tied: Sterilization and reproductive rights in America, 1950–1980.* Rutgers University Press.

Koerber, A. (2018). *From hysteria to hormones: A rhetorical history.* Penn State University Press.

Kopelson, K. (2019). Dying virtues: Medical doctors' epideictic rhetoric of how to die. *Rhetoric of Health & Medicine, 2*(3), 259–290.

LaVaque-Manty, Mika. (2017). Universalizing dignity in the nineteenth century. In R. Debes (Ed.), *Dignity: A history* (pp. 301–322). Oxford University Press.

Lemke, T. (2011). *Biopolitics: An advanced introduction* (E. F. Trump, Trans.). New York University Press.

Levinas, E. (1981). *Otherwise than being, or beyond essence* (Alphonso Lingis, Trans.). Springer Science & Business Media.

Lindner, E. G. (2001). Humiliation and human rights: Mapping a minefield. *Human Rights Review, 2*(2), 46–46.

Lipari, L. (2015). *Listening, thinking, being: Toward an ethics of attunement.* Penn State University Press.

Lorde, A. (2012). *Sister outsider: Essays and speeches.* Crossing Press.

Łuków, P. (2018). A difficult legacy: Human dignity as the founding value of human rights. *Human Rights Review, 19*(3), 313–329.

Lundberg, C., & Gunn, I. (2005). "Ouija board, are there any communications?" Agency, ontotheology, and the death of the humanist subject, or, continuing the ARS conversation. *Rhetoric Society Quarterly, 35*(4), 83–105.

Lynch, J. A. (2019). *The origins of bioethics: Remembering when medicine went wrong.* Michigan State University Press.

Macklin, R. (2003). Dignity is a useless concept. *BMJ, 327,* 1419.

Macready, J. D. (2018). *Hannah Arendt and the fragility of human dignity.* Lexington Books.

Malpas, J., & Lickiss, N. (Eds.). (2007). *Perspectives on human dignity: A conversation.* Springer Science & Business Media.

Manderson, L., Burke, N. J., & Wahlberg, A. (2021). *Viral loads: Anthropologies of urgency in the time of COVID-19.* UCL Press.

Mbembe, A. (2019) *Necropolitics.* Duke University Press.

McClellan, F. M. (2019). *Healthcare and human dignity: Law matters.* Rutgers University Press.

McCrudden, C. (2013). *Understanding human dignity.* Oxford University Press.

McDorman, T. F. (2005). Controlling death: Biopower and the right-to-die controversy. *Communication and Critical/Cultural Studies, 2*(3), 257–279.

McKittrick, K. (Ed.). (2015). *Sylvia Wynter: On being human as praxis.* Duke University Press.

McPherson, K., Gibson, B. E., & Leplège, A. (Eds.). (2015). *Rethinking rehabilitation: Theory and practice* (Vol. 10). CRC Press.

McRuer, R. (2010). Compulsory able-bodiedness and queer/disabled existence. In L. J. Davis (Ed.), *The Disability Studies Reader* (2nd ed., pp. 383–392). Routledge.

Menkiti, I. A. (1984). Person and community in African traditional thought. In R. Wright (Ed.), *African philosophy: An introduction* (pp. 171–182). University Press of America.

Meyer, M. A. (2001). Our own liberation: Reflections on Hawaiian epistemology. *Contemporary Pacific, 13*(1), 124–148.

Minear, A. (2011). "Unspeakable" offenses: Disability studies at the intersections of multiple differences. In N. Erevelles (Ed.), *Disability and difference in global contexts* (pp. 95–120). Palgrave Macmillan.

Mingus, M. (2011). Access intimacy: The missing link. *Leaving Evidence.* https://leavingevidence.wordpress.com/2011/05/05/access-intimacy-the-missing-link/

Mol, A. (2003). *The body multiple.* Duke University Press.

Mol, A. (2008). *The logic of care: Health and the problem of patient choice.* Routledge.

Mol, A. (2021). *Eating in theory.* Duke University Press.

Mol, A., Moser, I., & Pols, J. (Eds.). (2015). *Care in practice: On tinkering in clinics, homes and farms* (Vol. 8). transcript Verlag.

Molefe, M. (2018). Personhood and rights in an African tradition. *Politikon,* 45(2), 217–231.

Morris, J. (2020). *Human dignity: In (pragmatistic) defence of a (purportedly) useless concept* [Unpublished doctoral dissertation]. McMaster University.

Mosel, I., & Holloway, K. (2019). *Dignity and humanitarian action in displacement.* Humanitarian Policy Group, Overseas Development Institute. https://www.comminit.com/content/dignity-and-humanitarian-action-displacement

Muders, S. (Ed.). (2017). *Human dignity and assisted death.* Oxford University Press.

Murithi, T. (2007). A local response to the global human rights standard: The *ubuntu* perspective on human dignity. *Globalisation, Societies and Education,* 5(3), 277–286.

Murray, S. J. (2022). *The living from the dead: Disaffirming biopolitics.* Penn State University Press.

Nascimento, A., & Lutz-Bachmann, M. Human dignity in the perspective of a critical theory of human rights. In *Human dignity: Perspectives from a critical theory of human rights* (pp. 1–23). Routledge.

Neimanis, A. (2017). *Bodies of water: Posthuman feminist phenomenology.* Bloomsbury.

Nelson, A. (2011). *Body and soul: The Black Panther Party and the fight against medical discrimination.* University of Minnesota Press.

Nelson, J. (2003). *Women of color and the reproductive rights movement.* New York University Press.

Niccolini, A., & Ringrose, J. (2019). Feminist posthumanism. In P. A. Atkinson, S. Delamont, R. A. Williams, A. Cernat, & J. Sakshaug (Eds.), *SAGE research methods foundations.* Sage.

Nikolayenko, O. (2020). Invisible revolutionaries: Women's participation in the revolution of dignity. *Comparative Politics,* 52(3), 451–472.

Nussbaum, M. (2008). Human dignity and political entitlements. In *Human dignity and bioethics* (pp. 351–380). President's Council on Bioethics.

Nussbaum, M. C. (2019). *The cosmopolitan tradition.* Harvard University Press.

Oliver, M. (1992). Changing the social relations of research production? *Disability, Handicap & Society,* 7(2), 101–114.

Oliviero, K. (2018). *Vulnerability politics: The uses and abuses of precarity in political debate.* New York University Press.

Ornstein, K. A., Roth, D. L., Huang, J., Levitan, E. B., Rhodes, J. D., Fabius, C. D., Safford, M. M., & Sheehan, O. C. (2020). Evaluation of racial disparities in hospice use and end-of-life treatment intensity in the REGARDS cohort. *JAMA Network Open, 3*(8), e2014639–e2014639.

Örulv, L., & Nikku, N. (2007). Dignity work in dementia care: Sketching a microethical analysis. *Dementia, 6*(4), 507–525.

Patsavas, A. (2014). Recovering a cripistemology of pain. *Journal of Literary & Cultural Disability Studies, 8*(2), 203–219.

Phelps, L. W. (1991). Practical wisdom and the geography of knowledge in composition. *College English, 53*(8), 863–885.

Phillips, K. R. (1999). Tactical apologia: The American Nursing Association and assisted suicide. *Southern Journal of Communication, 64*(2), 143–154.

Pickering, A. (1993). The mangle of practice: Agency and emergence in the sociology of science. *American Journal of Sociology, 99*(3), 559–589.

Piepzna-Samarasinha, L. L. (2018). *Care work: Dreaming disability justice.* Arsenal Pulp Press.

Pols, J. (2006). Accounting and washing: Good care in long-term psychiatry. *Science, Technology & Human Values, 31*(4), 409–430.

Pols, J. (2013). Washing the patient: Dignity and aesthetic values in nursing care. *Nursing Philosophy, 14*(3), 186–200.

Pope, T. M. (2018). Legal history of medical aid in dying: Physician assisted death in the U.S. courts and legislatures. *New Mexico Law Review, 48*(2), 267–301.

Price, M. (2011). *Mad at school: Rhetorics of mental disability and academic life.* University of Michigan Press.

Price, M. (2015). The bodymind problem and the possibilities of pain. *Hypatia, 30*(1), 268–284.

Pringle, W. (2019). Problematizations in assisted dying discourse: Testing the "What's the problem represented to be?" (WPR) method for critical health communication research. *Frontiers in Communication, 4*(58), 1–11.

Puar, J. K. (2017). *The right to maim: Debility, capacity, disability.* Duke University Press.

Puig de la Bellacasa, M. (2017). *Matters of care: Speculative ethics in more than human worlds.* University of Minnesota Press.

Pullman, D. (2004). Death, dignity, and moral nonsense. *Journal of Palliative Care, 20*(3), 171–178.

Reynolds, J. M. (2022). *The life worth living: Disability, pain, and morality.* University of Minnesota Press.

Roberts, D. (1997). *Killing the black body: Race, reproduction, and the meaning of liberty.* Pantheon Books.

Rose, N. (2009). *The politics of life itself: Biomedicine, power, and subjectivity in the twenty-first century.* Princeton University Press.

Rosen, M. (2012). *Dignity: Its history and meaning.* Harvard University Press.

Rosiek, J. L., Snyder, J., & Pratt, S. L. (2020). The new materialisms and indigenous theories of non-human agency: Making the case for respectful anti-colonial engagement. *Qualitative Inquiry, 26*(3–4), 331–346.

Ross, L. J. (2017). Trust black women: Reproductive justice and eugenics. In L. J. Ross, L. Roberts, E. Derkas, W. Peoples, & P. B. Toure (Eds.), *Radical reproductive justice: Foundations, theory, practice, critique* (pp. 58–85). Feminist Press.

Rowntree, M. R. (2019). *Material intimacy: Bearing witness, listening, and wandering the ruins* [Unpublished doctoral dissertation]. University of Texas at Arlington.

Rusert, B. (2012). The science of freedom: Counterarchives of racial science on the antebellum stage. *African American Review, 45*(3), 291–308.

Saldaña, J. (2013). *The coding manual for qualitative researchers.* Sage.

Saldaña, J., & Omasta, M. (2022). *Qualitative research: Analyzing life.* Sage.

Schroeder, D., & Bani-Sadr, A. (2017). *Dignity in the 21st century: Middle east and west.* Springer.

Schryer, C., McDougall, A., Tait, G. R., & Lingard, L. (2012). Creating discursive order at the end of life: The role of genres in palliative care settings. *Written Communication, 29*(2), 111–141.

Schuster, M. L., Russell, A. L. B., Bartels, D. M., & Kelly-Trombley, H. (2013). "Standing in Terri Schiavo's shoes": The role of genre in end-of-life decision making. *Technical Communication Quarterly, 22*(3), 195–218.

Schuster, M. L., Russell, A. L., Bartels, D., & Kelly-Trombley, H. (2014). Determining "best interests" in end-of-life decisions for the developmentally disabled: Minnesota state guardians and wards. *Disability Studies Quarterly, 34*(4).

Scribner, S., & Cole, M. (1981). *The psychology of literacy.* Harvard University Press.

Scuro, J. (2017). *Addressing ableism: Philosophical questions via disability studies.* Lexington Books.

Segal, J. (2000a). What is a rhetoric of death? End-of-life decision-making at a psychiatric hospital. *Canadian Journal for Studies in Discourse and Writing, 16*(1), 65–86.

Segal, J. (2000b). Contesting death, speaking of dying. *Journal of Medical Humanities, 21*(1), 29–44.

Shershow, S. C. (2014). *Deconstructing dignity: A critique of the right-to-die debate.* University of Chicago Press.

Shildrick, M. (2009). *Dangerous discourses of disability, subjectivity and sexuality.* Springer.

Siebers, T. (2008). Disability experience on trial. In S. Alaimo & S. Hekman (Eds.), *Material Feminisms* (pp. 291–307). Indiana University Press.

Simplican, S. C. (2015). *The capacity contract: Intellectual disability and the question of citizenship.* University of Minnesota Press.

Snaza, N. (2020). Biopolitics without bodies: Feminism and the feeling of life. *Feminist Studies, 46*(1), 178–203.

Spivak, G. C. (2012). *An aesthetic education in the era of globalization.* Harvard University Press.

Stormer, N., & McGreavy, B. (2017). Thinking ecologically about rhetoric's ontology: Capacity, vulnerability, and resilience. *Philosophy & Rhetoric, 50*(1), 1–25.

Svendby, R., Romsland, G. I., & Moen, K. (2018). Non-disabled ableism: An autoethnography of cultural encounters between a non-disabled researcher and disabled people in the field. *Scandinavian Journal of Disability Research, 20*(1).

TallBear, K. (2013). *Native American DNA: Tribal belonging and the false promise of genetic science.* University of Minnesota Press.

Teston, C. (2017a). *Bodies in flux: Scientific methods for negotiating medical uncertainty.* University of Chicago Press.

Teston, C. (2017b). Enthymematic elasticity in the biomedical backstage. In L. Walsh & C. Boyle (Eds.), *Topologies as techniques for a post-critical rhetoric* (pp. 219–241). Palgrave Macmillan.

Teston, C. (2018). Pathologizing precarity. In W. S. Hesford, A. C. Licona, & C. Teston (Eds.), *Precarious rhetorics* (pp. 276–298). Ohio State University Press.

Teston, C., Gonzales, L., Bivens, K. M., & Whitney, K. (2019). Surveying precarious publics. *Rhetoric of Health & Medicine, 2*(3), 321–351.

Theobald, B. (2019). *Reproduction on the reservation: Pregnancy, childbirth, and colonialism in the long twentieth century.* University of North Carolina Press.

Tsing, A. L., Deger, J., Saxena, A. K., & Zhou, F. (Eds.). (2021). *Feral atlas: The more-than-human Anthropocene.* Stanford University Press [Online source]. https://feralatlas.org/

Van Der Graaf, R., & Van Delden, J. J. (2009). Clarifying appeals to dignity in medical ethics from an historical perspective. *Bioethics, 23*(3), 151–160.

Walsh, K., & Mignolo, W. (2018). *On decoloniality: Concepts, analytics, praxis.* Duke University Press.

Walsh, L., & Boyle, C. (2017). *Topologies as techniques for a post-critical rhetoric.* Springer.

Washington, H. A. (2006). *Medical apartheid: The dark history of medical experimentation on black Americans from colonial times to the present.* Doubleday Books.

Weber-Guskar, E. (2020). Deciding with dignity: The account of human dignity as an attitude and its implications for assisted suicide. *Bioethics, 34*(1), 135–141.

Weheliye, A. G. (2014). *Habeas viscus: Racializing assemblages, biopolitics, and black feminist theories of the human*. Duke University Press.

Wenger, E. (1998). *Communities of practice: Learning, meaning and identity*. Cambridge University Press.

Whatmore, S. (1997). Dissecting the autonomous self: Hybrid cartographies for a relational ethics. *Environment and Planning D: Society and Space, 15*, 37–53.

Wiggermann, N., Zhou, J., & Kumpar, D. (2020). Proning patients with COVID-19: A review of equipment and methods. *Human Factors, 62*(7), 1069–1076.

Willey, A. (2016). *Undoing monogamy: The politics of science and the possibilities of biology*. Duke University Press.

Williamson, B. (2019). *Accessible America*. New York University Press.

Willis, R. (2019). The use of composite narratives to present interview findings. *Qualitative Research, 19*(4), 471–480.

Woodward, K. (2004). Calculating compassion. In L. Berlant (Ed.), *Compassion: The culture and politics of an emotion* (pp. 59–86). Routledge.

Wynter, S. (1994). "No humans involved": An open letter to my colleagues. *Forum N.H.I.: Knowledge for the 21st Century, 1*(1), 1–17.

Wynter, S. (2003). Unsetting the coloniality of being/power/truth/freedom: Towards the human, after man, its overrepresentation—an argument. *New Centennial Review, 3*(3), 257–337.

Yam, S. S. (2020). Visualizing birth stories from the margin: Toward a reproductive justice model of rhetorical analysis. *Rhetoric Society Quarterly, 50*(1), 19–34.

Yergeau, M. R. (2018). *Authoring autism: On rhetoric and neurological queerness*. Duke University Press.

Young, I. M. (1997). *Intersecting voices: Dilemmas of gender, political philosophy, and policy*. Princeton University Press.

Zemlicka, K. (2013). The rhetoric of enhancing the human: Examining the tropes of "the human" and "dignity" in contemporary bioethical debates over enhancement technologies. *Philosophy & Rhetoric, 46*(3), 257–279.

INDEX